Reichian Bodywork

Melting the blocks to life and love

Second Edition

Nick Totton
and
Em Edmondson

Illustrated by Kirsty O'Connor

PCCS BOOKS
Monmouth

PCCS BOOKS
Wyatsone Business Park
Wyastone Leys
MONMOUTH
NP25 3SR
UK
Tel +44 (0)1600 891509

www.pccs-books.co.uk

This edition published 2009

First edition published 1988
by Prism Press

Text © Nick Totton and Em Edmondson, 2009
Illustrations © Kirsty O'Connor, 2009

All rights reserved.
No part of this publication may be reproduced, stored in
a retrieval system, transmitted or utilised in any form by
any means, electronic, mechanical, photocopying or
recording or otherwise without permission in writing
from the publishers.

Nick Totton and Em Edmondson have asserted their rights
to be identified as the authors of this work in accordance with the
Copyright, Designs and Patents Act 1988.

Reichian Growth Work
Melting the blocks to life and love

ISBN 978-1-906254-12-4

Cover design in the UK by Old Dog Graphics
Cover photographs provided by Nick Totton (front) and Em Edmondson (back)
Typeset in the UK by The Old Dog's Missus in 'Univers'
Printed in the UK by ImprintDigital, Exeter.

Contents

	Introduction	1
Chapter 1	Contexts	6
Chapter 2	Energy and Armour	11
Chapter 3	Surrender	21
Chapter 4	The Segments	28
Chapter 5	Growing Up	55
Chapter 6	Character Positions	65
Chapter 7	More on Character	86
Chapter 8	Therapy	96
Chapter 9	Power	118
Chapter 10	Primal Patterns	125
Chapter 11	Cosmic Streaming	133
Chapter 12	Connections and Directions	141
	Further Reading	149
	Index	161

For the children
Jo, Zoë, Jacob and Mica

Introduction to the Second Edition

CHANGING AND STAYING THE SAME

The first edition of this book was published twenty years ago; since then it has appeared in Dutch, Italian and Spanish versions. Thinking about this new English edition, two things in particular have struck us: how much the context in which we are working has changed – and how little, in essence, our own thinking has changed.

Of course our own thinking and practice have developed a great deal over those two decades. We have absorbed many new ideas and approaches, and learnt a lot more about existing ones. Also, our style of work has generally *broadened:* we have taken on the fact that different people need different things from therapy, and that it is not very helpful to try to make clients fit our way of doing things – instead, we have to be able to meet them where they are.

When we say that the essence of our thinking has not changed greatly, we mean that we still see the world and human beings in much the same way that we outline in this book. We still approach therapy as a way of helping people to *relax*, to let go of the patterns of bodily/emotional tension which they have adopted as protection from the demands of society and from painful experience in general, and to allow their own spontaneous self-expression. Our understanding of *how* to do this has of course developed a great deal! Some of these new understandings are covered in this second edition, and in the Further Reading at the end, including other books by Nick which are mentioned there.

So what has changed in the context of our work? Looking back, when the first edition was published we were working pretty much in isolation, in a little Yorkshire post-Reichian bubble. We knew very little about most other forms even of Reichian work, let alone of psychotherapy in general, and we knew very few practitioners outside our own approach. There were a lot fewer practitioners around of course – this was the mid 1980s, and since then the scale of therapy and counselling in this country has increased out of all recognition.

Along with this has come a whole new climate around therapy, a concern about evidence, effectiveness and regulation. Large organisations and institutions have evolved, claiming to protect clients but in reality perhaps more concerned with establishing their own power base. After many years of lobbying, these organisations have succeeded in achieving the regulation of therapy and counselling – unfortunately for them, though, not on the basis they envisaged, which would have put them in control of the therapy world. Instead, state regulation will probably mean that existing organisations become superfluous; what will happen instead is, at the point of writing, impossible to predict.

In this new atmosphere of regulation and control, the sort of work which this book describes has in some ways become more shocking and suspicious to many people. At the same time, interestingly enough, it has also achieved new recognition and interest, after a partial eclipse during the 1990s. These days, everyone is talking about embodiment and about body psychotherapy; some people are even looking for hands-on work with breath and energy. It seems as though a swing of the pendulum towards the mainstream has produced a simultaneous swing in the opposite direction, towards ideas and approaches that challenge mainstream attitudes and ways of behaving.

When embodiment is discussed in the therapy world today, it is usually linked with two concepts which we did not even mention in the first edition, because although virtually omnipresent now, they were scarcely on the horizon at that time. These are *attachment* and *trauma*. We have included a section on trauma in this new edition, near the end of Chapter 2, where we try to make clear that although Reich does not use the word, the idea of trauma is close to the heart of his thinking. We have also included some relevant further reading on this topic at the end of the book.

Attachment is trickier: John Bowlby's attachment theory is based on very different assumptions from Reichian work, and it is not clear that the two are really compatible. Reich was deeply committed to an *energetic* model of human existence, in which life energy gives rise to desire of all kinds, what Freud called 'libido', and the work of therapy is to re-establish the free flow of this energy. This is the viewpoint we take in this book. Attachment theory, by contrast, is centred on the infant–carer relationship, seen as biologically hardwired; it understands the sorts of problems which bring people into therapy to be largely about disturbances of attachment in early childhood.

Any unbiased person looking at these two sets of ideas is likely to feel that both have some truth to them. However, it is not that easy to make them fit together intellectually. Perhaps this is not too important, at any rate for now: body psychotherapy seems to be going through a 'paradigm shift', out of which a new synthesis of these two models will hopefully emerge. One of Reich's statements suggests a way forward: 'There is but one desire which issues from the biopsychic unity of the person,' he says, 'the desire to discharge inner tensions. This is impossible without contact with the outer world. Hence, the *first* impulse of *every* creature must be the desire to establish contact with the outer world.'

Attachment and trauma are both associated with the extraordinary new discoveries of neuroscience, many of which have been taken up enthusiastically by therapists and counsellors. No one is keener on this than body psychotherapists, largely because neuroscience research has confirmed many of our strongest beliefs in the most precise and uncanny way. This is shown by the fact that, although none of this research was known at the time we wrote the first edition, this has not meant that we have needed to make any substantial changes. Some of the most important writing on the topic is listed at the end of the book.

The key thing for us about this book is that it is not aimed primarily at therapists, but at ordinary people with an interest in self-development. Some of the positive feedback we have received from non-therapists over the years has been a great source of pride. As time goes on there appear to be fewer and fewer books which describe therapy in a serious way, but in ordinary language and short sentences. Therapy, it seems, has become a subject for therapists only, too technical for the 'lay person'. We vehemently disagree. If people are going to be empowered by therapy, then they need to be able to understand what it is about, what it is trying to achieve and how it goes about it.

THE NEW EDITION

We have already mentioned some of the alterations to this edition, but now we want to talk about them more systematically. If you have not read the first edition then you may want to skip the next few paragraphs.

We made a decision early on not to write a completely new book: we think that the existing book is essentially sound, and also a significant historical document. Nick has summed up his more recent ideas in several other books and articles, some of which are listed under Further Reading, and in general we have used that section as an alternative to rewriting the whole book, listing as many as possible of the important works that have appeared since 1986.

We have, however, made quite a lot of changes to the original text, and these are of three kinds. First, we have taken the opportunity to clarify and develop many of the points we tried to make in the first edition – everything from changing a particular word to adding a couple of paragraphs – partly just to improve the writing, but also to incorporate later ideas of our own and other people's. Secondly, overall we have softened the tone of our writing, making it less dogmatic and absolute, and emphasising people's individuality and the need to meet each person where they are.

Thirdly, we have added a certain amount of new material. As already mentioned, there is a section on trauma. The other, very important change is that we have added a character position which was not present in the first edition: the Control character. There is some controversy about this character position in the Reichian world, but we have become convinced that it is not only real, but highly important, being based on the heart and the extent of its openness or closedness. In order to include this character a lot of Chapters 6 and 7 have been revised.

As well as adding this character, we have dropped the idea of the Open character which we included in the original book. This was included partly in homage to Reich's vision of the 'genital character', but we have come to realise that the idea of a 'correct', 'healthy' character position goes against everything we are trying to say in this book, so we have rewritten the section talking about relative and temporary states of openness and armouredness.

The new edition retains the splendid illustrations provided for the original edition by Kirsty O'Connor.

OURSELVES

So what has happened to us over the last twenty years? Well, we have grown older. We are both still working as therapists, but no longer working or living together. Nick has written a number of books about body psychotherapy, psychotherapy and politics, and other topics; he has also published his collected poems. He lives in Calderdale, West Yorkshire. Em has trained in Hakomi therapy, and become a certified trainer; she has also trained in Authentic Movement. She has a house on the west coast of Ireland, but still lives mainly in Leeds. Both of us have learnt a lot more about psychoanalytic ideas, and also about Arnold Mindell's Process Work.

From these styles of work we have learnt many things. In particular we now have a deeper understanding of the need to respect and support where a person *is* rather than trying to move them to where we think they *should* be. We feel that this approach was already implicit in the original book, but now we would go further in rejecting the 'making better, putting right' approach to therapy. What needs to happen is already trying to happen; it only requires a little help.

Learning about psychoanalysis – which was of course where Reich himself was rooted – has enriched and deepened our grasp of Reichian therapy; in particular, it has strengthened the emphasis in our work on relationship between client and practitioner. We would now formulate the central question of Reichian bodywork as: How can I breathe and relate at the same time?

We both feel less optimistic than we did in 1986. As one grows older, one has to accept on a personal level that possibilities are limited, and some dreams will never be realised. The world also seems a grimmer and more fragile place, and there is nowhere to stand to get the perspective which will tell us whether this too is the product of ageing, or whether it is objectively true. Certainly the ecological disaster which one could already sense in the 1980s – and which Reich himself foretold in the 1950s – is now fully upon us, and no one knows how far into catastrophe we will have to go before we are able to change our path as a society, nor what price non-human species will have to pay for our folly.

But life persists; hope persists. Life energy will always seek a way to fulfil itself; for us, that is one of the most profound lessons we have learnt from our work as therapists. As we said in the introduction to the first edition, this book is for people who want to change; because only by changing, profoundly painful as that sometimes is, can we stay alive and growing.

1

Contexts

> Nobody knows
> how it flows
> as it goes
> Nobody goes
> where it rose
> where it flows
> Nobody chose
> how it grows
> how it flows
>
> Marge Piercy, *Woman on the Edge of Time*

In this book we describe a form of therapeutic work with groups and individuals which derives originally from the work of Wilhelm Reich, but also from a number of other developments in therapy and healing, especially since Reich's death in 1957. It is the style in which we, the authors, were trained, but which we have also developed in new directions.

Although Reichian therapy has always attracted great interest – and still does – there is very little written about it that is useful for the ordinary reader. Some of Reich's own books are inspiring and moving, but those on the therapy itself and the theory behind it are very technical and hard to follow, aimed at an audience of medically trained psychoanalysts. They are also very dated in relation to the sort of work actually being done at present.

In writing this book, we have tried to avoid jargon as far as possible. New words are sometimes needed to describe new ideas and experiences, but we have defined each of these clearly when it first appears, and remind you of its meaning when we use it again. More generally, we have tried never to use a long word when a short one will do. We have written for the sort of people who, we find, are interested in the work we do, many of whom are by no stretch of the imagination intellectuals. The new interest in therapy and growth work is part of a very broadly based concern with *change*, both on an individual and on a social level. Many people in our society are deeply dissatisfied with their conditions of life, and more and more of them are no longer willing to be the sort of person that society expects and forces them to be – mentally, emotionally, spiritually, even physically.

This book is for people who want to change.

WHO REICH WAS

If you want to know about Reich's life and work, several books are listed under 'Further Reading' at the end of the book. In brief, Wilhelm Reich (1897–1957) as a young man trained with Freud in Vienna, and worked as a psychoanalyst. Besides making some important advances in technique, he soon 'burst the bounds' of psychoanalysis, moving into a deeper confrontation both with the clients themselves, and with the social conditions which he saw as creating and maintaining their problems.

An energetic, combative and challenging man, Reich managed in a few short years to attract the enmity of the Nazis, the Communist Party (of which he was a member for several years), and the psychoanalytic establishment. As he travelled around Scandinavia and eventually to the USA as a refugee from the Nazis, he managed to achieve some fundamental breakthroughs in therapeutic methods; in particular, he created the whole new field of bodywork.

Reich became increasingly focused on life energy itself, and on finding ways to unblock, condense, channel and strengthen that energy, both in the human body and in the atmosphere. Above all, Reich was a person with open eyes: he noticed a lot of things which most people prefer to ignore, and this led him into many exciting new areas of enquiry – and attracted a lot of hostility.

As well as giving therapy to individuals, and becoming involved with the healthy upbringing of children, Reich created devices like the 'orgone accumulator' (to concentrate life energy) and the 'cloudbuster' (with which he believed he could affect pollution and weather). He became acutely sensitive to oppressive conditions in the physical and social atmosphere, and struggled to find ways of combating these 'plagues'.

At the same time, Reich continued to come up against anger and aggression, very largely because of his open and celebratory approach to sex, which got him into hot water throughout his life. In the last few years of Reich and his circle, there was a steady 'darkening', a distortion of feelings and perceptions, which derived at least partly from a disastrous 'Oranur' experiment using orgone accumulators to try to neutralise radiation, but also from the constant pressure of both outside enemies and internal disciples.

Finally, Reich was prosecuted by the US federal authorities, accused – quite falsely – of peddling his accumulators as a fake cancer cure. Reich could almost certainly have won the case if he had fought on legal grounds: instead he refused to recognise the court's jurisdiction over 'issues of scientific truth'. The legal system in turn saw Reich as an awkward, suspect foreign crackpot; he was jailed for contempt, and died in prison of a heart attack shortly before he was due for release. His accumulators were destroyed and his books burned by the American government.

Using Reich's techniques and reading his books, it is sometimes hard not to fall into discipleship. He was a person of extraordinary perceptions, and of great compassion and courage: a big-hearted man. He was also, clearly, an extremely awkward customer, and someone who expected to get his own way. He also had his own hang-ups – an anti-homosexual stance, for example, with which we very strongly disagree.

WHO WE ARE

We live together in Leeds with our young baby daughter and with Em's son. We both work as therapists and group leaders, moving into this work through doing a training in Reichian therapy led by William West. This training, which finished in 1982, was only the beginning. As we started to work with clients, we found much that we didn't know, and searched out ways of learning it, through books, through further training, and through talking out our experiences together and with other people.

A result of that first Reichian training led by William was the creation of 'Energy Stream: the Post Reichian Therapy Association'. Three training courses later – one led by William, two by ourselves – Energy Stream includes some thirty practising therapists, all working in their own personal style and with a range of techniques, but all sharing the same commitment to Reichian work.

We talk about 'Reichian work', but what is it? There are many approaches which could claim a right to that label. During his career Reich worked differently at different times, and there are several schools of therapy descended from people he trained in various ways. There are also several schools developed after Reich's death which have consciously changed his ideas and methods; many of these call themselves 'neo-Reichian'.

We see our own work as very close to the essence of Reich's, but not everyone would agree with us. We certainly don't know whether Reich would agree with us! We sometimes like to think that he might be working in this sort of way if he was still alive, but there are many things we do of which he strongly disapproved. So this book is about *our* work, and not, either, specifically about Energy Stream's methods. However, we are very grateful to everyone in Energy Stream for their support, stimulation and encouragement, especially William West who originally trained us and gave us therapy; Annie Morgan, Rika Petersen and Sean Doherty, who helped lead the last training course; Mary Swale; and Holly Clutterbuck, Maxine Higham and Pam Wilkinson, with whom Nick sorted out many of these ideas in a supervision group.

This book is not intended to be a manual for therapists – although we hope it will be useful for therapists. It is aimed mainly at anyone trying to change, searching for ideas about how to change, about how we are and why we are like that. We are writing about 'human nature', human beings as part of nature, as natural beings. It is for a vision of *naturalness*, above all, that we thank Reich, and it is in pursuit of naturalness (which ultimately cannot be pursued) that we have learnt from and adapted many other ways of perceiving and working with people. Thank you to everyone who has helped us learn.

We want to make it very clear that in writing a book about therapy we are not claiming to be 'super shrinks'. Still less are we claiming to be totally clear, enlightened individuals who have sorted out all our problems. Anyone who knows us would find such an idea laughable. We felt that the book needed writing, and we felt able to do it. Now we have to go on trying to live up to these ideas.

You may notice that there are no case histories included in this book. It's always good fun to read about a therapist's clients and their sessions, as good as a novel, and in some ways it is very informative. But it is also very easy – in fact, inevitable – to oversimplify the wholeness of a person's life and struggle. We felt that any of our clients would be bound to recognise themselves, and that this sort of thumbnail sketch would be disrespectful to their courage and complexity. However, all our clients do of course feature in these pages, and we want to thank them as well, together with those who have attended our workshops, and especially those whom we have trained. There could be no book without you.

Our method of collaboration on the book has been for Nick (the verbally oriented one) to write chunks of it and show them to Em (the feeling oriented one), who has read them and explained to Nick how no ordinary person could make head or tail of it all. Nick then went away and re-wrote until it passed the test. Of course, we don't always agree on every detail, and some of what follows reflects more the views of one or other of us. But to a remarkable extent we do agree about people and therapy (after all, it was through Reichian therapy that we met in the first place).

Meanwhile our own work moves on. Like the rest of Energy Stream, we have other interests, other skills. We have recently formed a separate identity, 'Selfheal', as a vehicle for the whole of our healing work, including but not restricted to the 'Reichian' element. This doesn't mean that we have turned our backs on anything we describe in this book, simply that the stream goes on flowing, broadening and deepening, meeting with other streams, merging into a greater river, on the way to the sea.

We hope that what follows helps *you* to flow.

2

Energy and Armour

Our feelings and our bodies are like water flowing into water. We learn to swim within the energies of the senses.

    Tarthang Tulku, *Kum Nye Relaxation*

He who remains passive when overwhelmed with grief loses his best chance of recovering elasticity of mind.

    Charles Darwin, *The Expression of the Emotions in Man and Animals*

LIFE HAS ENERGY

Or rather, life *is* energy: moving, vibrating, seeking, pulsing. We may not be able to define life energy, but we all experience it in our own beings, and perceive it in other people: watching a fine dancer or mime or T'ai Chi exponent, making love, meditating, expressing strong emotion, receiving or giving hands-on healing. Many people over the ages have given names to the life energy and its different forms – 'prana', 'magnetic fluid', 'vital essence', 'chi', 'od', 'archeus', 'kundalini', and many more. Reich's name for it was 'Orgone', which he made up from words like 'orgasm' and 'organism'.

    This life energy is the vitality of our being: when we are moved, this is what moves. Emotions are 'e-motions', movements out; they are not just in our minds, but in our bodies, in the charge of energy that builds up and with luck, discharges; in the flooding of hormones, the surge of bodily fluids and electrical potential, expanding from deep within us towards the surface, or retreating into the caves of the abdomen, or flowing through and out via head and hands and legs and pelvis, shifting form easily between muscular or electrical tension, fluid, sound, movement sensation, emotion.

    For example: I feel sorrow, but am inhibited about showing it. So as it 'rises' in me, maybe my throat contracts – I'm 'all choked up', mucus forms and my throat aches; my chin tightens and tucks in as part of the effort to restrict flow in my neck; maybe my fists tense, and transmit that 'holding' up my arms to my shoulders and throat – I'm 'keeping a grip on myself'.

If my grief starts to break through the holding, probably I'll first sigh, cough or groan, release what I'm 'swallowing down' in the form of sound or mucus. As a channel opens up, a sensation of softening and melting flows up the sides of my throat and jaw. Another person can actually watch my cheeks suffuse with fluid and colour, my face softening as the emotion ex-presses (pushes out) through my eyes in the form of tears, with the piercing sweetness of release. At the same time my hands will open, my shoulders come forward in a vulnerable 'giving' gesture as my chest heaves with sobs, my 'full heart melts'. As I surrender physically to my grief, my mind may fill with corresponding thoughts, memories and images.

Thoughts, emotions, sensations, changes in electrolytic fluid, muscle tension, connective tissue, hormone balance, and flow of life energy: there is no point in saying that any one of these causes or comes before the others. They are different aspects of a single whole event in a single whole bodymind. We will focus on one or other of these aspects depending on what we are trying to find out or do.

Focusing on the play of life energy has the advantage of being fresh and uncompromised by our society's dubious assumptions about what feelings are. It gives the space to include many different aspects of the bodymind. It's a good starting point, but we don't want to give the impression that we think energy 'causes' thoughts, feelings or bodily changes. There is only the endless dance of transformation.

In fact we are all used to speaking about ourselves in energy images. These metaphors are often very literal, as when we say we feel full of energy, or drained and empty; our head is whirling or stuffed up; we feel electric; someone else is magnetically attractive; we have itchy feet; we melt with desire.

If we look at the human being as an *organism* among other organisms, to see what it shares with the rest of life, from amoebae to elephants, then we will almost certainly notice the role of *pulsation*. Life is constantly expanding and shrinking, reaching out and pulling back in response to internal needs and to outside influences – the 'friendliness' or 'hostility' of the environment. These continuous wavelike vibrations are the organism's ongoing 'conversation' with the rest of the universe. In humans, one expression of this continuous pulsing is our heartbeat, sending oxygenated blood out to the extremities of the organism and bringing waste products back. Another is the pulsing of cerebrospinal fluid – the craniosacral rhythm. Another, and particularly important for our purpose, is the *breath*.

> **Exercise 1**
> As you read what follows, and other passages later on, notice your bodily and emotional reactions. You will probably be stirred, as your own body memories are stimulated; but this often goes on outside our conscious awareness – which is one of the big themes of this book! See whether you can be aware of changes in your breath, tension, and emotions, and of how your bodily and emotional charge rises and falls as you read.

Watch a small baby breathe, and you'll see how the whole of her body is involved, committed, swept up in the smooth wavelike expansion and contraction that reaches from top to toes. For the healthy baby there's no resistance, no avoidance of the involuntary breath-pulse; at the top of the outbreath the inbreath is born and the top of the inbreath turns out again, Yin from Yang and Yang from Yin, a constant exchange of polarities with the universe (Yin and Yang are ancient Chinese names for the two complementary poles of existence, the Active and the Receptive).

As we grow up and confront this difficult world however, a *voluntary* element soon creeps into our breathing, a hesitation, a holding back, which likewise affects our whole body from top to toes. Inbreath and outbreath begin to separate from each other, to lose their seamless continuity, to become more shallow and jerky, without the generous graceful flow. We may develop a tendency to constantly hold our breath, never fully emptying our lungs or, contrariwise, to keep our lungs permanently half empty. And so we lose our basic grounding in the universe, our sense that we rise out of it and are of the same substance as it. We become separate, lost, lonely, anxious beings.

Why does this happen? If we *breathe* freely and fully, then we *feel* freely and fully. Open breathing washes emotion through and out into expression; we are unable to hide it, either from ourselves or from each other. Yet from a very early age, most of us experience a need to suppress some of our feelings.

This is because our environment – initially mainly the adults who are caring for us – does not support us in our feelings. They reject our neediness or tears or anger. They threaten us with punishment – including the withdrawal of love. Or they simply do not give the validation and care which our baby-self needs in order to cope with powerful feelings. This process can begin at birth or even sooner, as we shall see. It's no one's *fault*, generally speaking; all of us who are parents know how our own anxiety and pain and practical problems interfere with the sincere wish to nurture our children. But the *effect* is that children learn to hold back on feeling – by holding back on its expression – by holding back on breathing.

Don't worry if you are finding this difficult to follow (this might partly be because it is stirring to read about). We'll be coming back to this theme over and over again. But to make it a little more concrete, consider two examples. Imagine a baby who cries out as her natural way of expressing a need – hunger, cold, a desire for company – and no one comes. It will take a long time for this to sink in: she will cry and cry again, but eventually she will stop. She suppresses her crying by holding her breath – which holds back her grief and anger, not identified consciously as *feelings*, but implicit in the whole state of her body. Now imagine another baby who is picked up and manipulated by cold hands: not so much physically cold, but *emotionally* cold, uncaring. Babies feel these things, and there will be a reaction of shock, a gasp, like the way we gasp if we step into cold water. If this experience of cold touch is repeated often enough, then that gasp, that held breath, will become built in to the baby's body nature.

These are only examples from among many ways in which an unfriendly environment can interrupt the full, whole-body, involuntary pulsation of natural breathing. Muscles tense against it, first in the diaphragm, which is our primary breathing muscle (see Chapter 4), and then spreading into the chest, throat, back, belly, pelvis, arms and legs, face, head. The entire body is drawn into a battle against itself, against its own natural impulse to breathe and feel. In effect the energy 'splits', turns back on itself and blocks its own natural movement, like Indian wrestling with ourselves. The basic pattern of the diagram below is one that Reich used repeatedly, applying it to different situations.

Life energy splits and fights itself

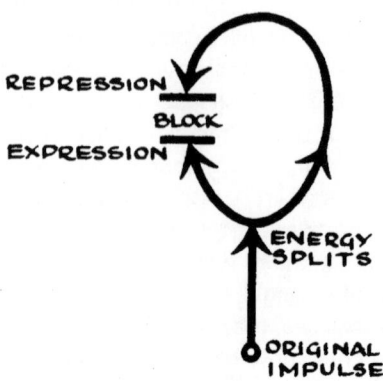

Energy and Armour 15

Sometimes the battle is conscious – whenever we deliberately tighten our jaw, tense our belly, swallow down emotion. But the infant's basic holding back against breathing quite soon becomes unconscious. If you think about it, this must happen: the purpose of the holding is precisely to stop us feeling our feelings, and this can only work if it stops us knowing what our feelings are. Emotions are bodily events; if they are blocked in the body, then they don't happen in the mind either. The fundamental holding acts as a *pattern* around which every later denial of feeling organises itself; we get very good at it indeed, artists and technicians of self-deception and self-denial.

> **Exercise 2**
> Take a moment now to check out how you are feeling and breathing. It's very likely that, while reading the above, you've tightened yourself up to resist the inward stirring these ideas create. So first put your attention in your belly and diaphragm – all around your navel, above and below. Is it gently rising and falling with your breath; or have you been holding it rigid? Are you able to deliberately relax it and let the tension flow out – perhaps with a sigh or a groan to help it along? Check out whether your chest, too, moves as you breathe – as part of a continuous wavelike flow with your belly. If not, you are probably holding your shoulders, hands, and/or jaw stiff. Try to let them go, and experience the feeling they have been holding on to. Allow yourself to breathe easily and fully; just watch where the holding is, if anywhere, and what thoughts cause an interruption to the flow. As you go on reading, try to come back periodically to a conscious awareness of your own breath and body state.

Blocked breathing is the essence of *armouring*: Reich's name for the state of chronic muscle tension and emotional holding back by which almost all adults in our society are imprisoned. Along with the suppression of breathing goes the suppression of specific impulses – to cry, to yell, to laugh, to hit, to reach out for love, to run away. The muscles are tightened to stop us e-moting, moving out, and if this tightening happens regularly enough it becomes a chronic, unconscious habit, built into the structure of our bodies – part of our sense of ourselves, as familiar as an old scar.

(Reich's basic idea of armouring was about muscular tension, and armouring does indeed often manifest as rigidity. However, there are other patterns as well: for example, a deep muscular holding can underlie what on the surface appears as placidity or softness. And sometimes someone learns to under-use particular groups of muscles, to keep them flaccid rather than tense. But don't worry too much about the details for now, stay with the central idea of muscular armouring.)

In fact, a lot of what we customarily identify as a person's 'self' is really their pattern of armouring: their high, tight shoulders, or stuck-out chest, or pulled-back jaw, or wide-open or narrowed-down eyes, or collapsed, defeated posture. 'Well, that's just the way I am,' they'll say. But in fact it's the way that person has *become*, by cutting off certain forms of self-expression and emphasising others.

Maybe one individual is constantly angry and aggressive, never letting herself feel soft, sad and small. Another is continuously polite and meek, censoring any assertiveness. As we shall see later, there are specific relationships between muscular armouring and emotional armouring: these cut-off emotions are locked into tense muscle patterns, locked in permanent, frozen battle with the suppressing impulses. They are imprisoned there like genies, bottled up in the rigid 'no' of our bodies. And, like genies, they can often be released by rubbing! – perhaps a direct physical stimulus, or perhaps in verbal or emotional form like supportive attention, stroking more than rubbing.

Our held-in feelings have *power*. When we liberate a feeling we can liberate not only the energy of the feeling itself, but also the split-off energy that has been devoted to holding it down. In doing this, we allow our breathing to open up, drawing on the infinite energy of the universe around us.

THE 'SPASTIC I'

Unfortunately this empowering process has a frightening side to it. It also involves releasing the fear of consequences which made us shut down our feeling in the first place: the fear of adult anger or coldness or withdrawal, the fear of a dangerous universe. Even more, it means changing the whole basis of our identity – the sense of 'I' upon which our life is founded. Opening up can sometimes seem like a threat to our very survival.

As Freud pointed out, our sense of 'I' (he used the German *Ich*, though it was translated into English with the Latin word *Ego*) starts out in the *body*. As the infant grows, she begins to organise bodily sensations and impulses into a whole, to 'take command' of them and develop an image of 'me' – when she looks in the mirror she realises that this image is herself, that this is how other people see her. In a healthy and supportive situation, she can grow into a powerful, realistic capacity for self-management, based on a strong but relaxed sense of identity and wholeness.

Tragically, our culture doesn't generally let this process of self-management happen naturally in its own time and rhythm. Many children are fed and put to bed and toilet-trained to fit in with the needs and timetables of adults. They are often forced with threats to bring processes like excretion under rigid control when this should be developing spontaneously. Small children literally *cannot* control their anal sphincters: the muscle–nerve connections aren't formed. So they must tense up the whole pelvic floor in a massive, straining effort to 'hold it in', a tension which easily becomes chronic, extending to the whole body and tightening the breath, so that the person 'holds themselves in' on every level.

Other children have a very different experience; they are not held and supported by the sorts of structures they need in order to learn self-management. The adults around them are too chaotic, depressed or self-centred to offer them bed times, toilet training and other useful boundaries. They will also armour themselves against the fear that this *lack* of holding brings.

Similarly, if our feeding is controlled by timetable, or if we are forced to eat food we don't like or not fed properly at all, then we 'swallow' an external controlling or ignoring of our bodily processes, and have to swallow down our rage if we want to get fed at all. These are all examples of the way in which the whole business of attaining self-management in our own body, which can be a proud and joyful affirmation of autonomy, very easily gets entangled with patterns of denial and negation, so that our very sense of 'I' is bound up with bodily tension. Like boys at an old-fashioned public school, we learn to 'get a grip on ourselves', and to *identify* with that grip. Feeling tense becomes part of our continuous background experience, so that full relaxation seems like a threat to our existence, as if we are going to melt and drain away completely.

Exercise 3

Breathe in, and deliberately tighten your non-dominant hand (the one that you don't write with) into a clenched fist. Hold it for as long as you comfortably can; then let your breath out, and let your fist relax. Notice the sensations while clenching, and when relaxing. Now breathe in and try to 'clench' your whole body in the same way; let your breath out and relax. Notice the sensations and emotions. Is there any part of your body that doesn't want to relax?

Just as muscles are forced into chronic spasm in order to comply with external restrictions or abandonment rather than inner self-regulation, so our 'I' develops a 'spastic', uncontrollably rigid emotional tone – a set of fixed attitudes towards the world and other people which we are unable to vary in response to changing circumstances. The 'I' becomes identical with the body armour.

'Armouring' is a good name for this process of physical and emotional rigidification. Muscle armour, like its medieval counterpart, is hard, stiff, restrictive, suffocating; also like iron armour, its original purpose was *defence*. We have no reason to feel guilty and inadequate about being armoured; on the contrary, it represents our skill and courage to survive in very difficult circumstances.

We have always done the best we can, making a rational decision to protect our vulnerable insides from an unsafe world – and, since we're still here, we have succeeded! But the price has been high in lost pleasure and potential. Now that we are bigger and stronger we have the option of melting our armour, re-experiencing our feelings in a safer way – and letting our soft pink insides out to play in the sunshine!

Of course, even now there isn't always sunshine; it isn't always safe or appropriate to be soft. People often get the idea that Reichian-type therapy will leave them vulnerable to whatever comes along. But the whole aim is to regain the power to choose, the power to be loving and open, or to scorch with righteous rage, or to close off totally for a while. Very few of us have access to the whole range of possible reactions.

Another way in which muscular armouring resembles its iron counterpart is that it tends to be arranged in *segments:* bands of tension that wrap horizontally round the body, constricting flow along the head-to-feet axis. If you imagine how a worm or snake moves, in wavy pulses, this gives a good image of the free unarmoured body. But if something pins the serpent down at one point in its length, the graceful undulation turns into jerking and thrashing.

This is like a human body becoming armoured in one segment: it can no longer expand and pulse in a smooth, expressive, unified way – expression becomes distorted and ugly, both physically and emotionally.

Most of us are armoured in more than one place. It's as if the snake is a child's wooden toy, split up into separate stiff lengths and able to bend only at the joints between the segments, in a parody of undulation. Having lost our sense of unity with the world through disjointed breathing, we lose our sense of *internal* unity through the disjointing effects of the armouring.

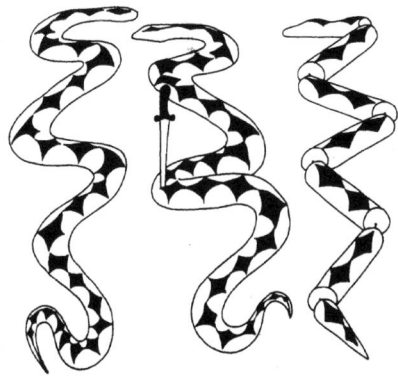

We'll look in much more detail later on at the segments and what they mean, but it's worth emphasising here that the specific details of armouring, as Reich described them or as we use them doing therapy – so many segments in such and such places – are rules of thumb rather than gospel truth. The human organism is immensely rich and complex, full of subtle channels, links, patterns and mirrorings, and each human individual is in many ways unique.

But the more each of us is armoured, the less freedom of expression we have, the less individuality and richness; and the more we tend to operate in a groove to correspond to the mechanical system of the segments. It's the *armouring* that has segments, not the person, and the process of therapy is precisely one of rediscovering our individual uniqueness.

TRAUMA

These issues are now most commonly discussed in terms of 'traumatisation'. 'Trauma' is the Ancient Greek word for 'wound'; and therapists have long understood that psychological wounds can have just as long-lasting and damaging effects as physical ones.

More recently, neuroscientists have explored the physical aspect of psychological wounding: the long-term effects that it can have on our nervous system, conditioning our ability to feel, think, relate and generally operate effectively in the world. Much of what they have discovered confirms the intuition and experience of Reich and other body psychotherapists in the most striking way.

However, Reich was mainly concerned with the effects not of shattering one-off trauma – important though that is – but of what one might call chronic, everyday, sub-acute trauma: the cumulative impact of being brought up in emotionally toxic environments, without the sort of loving and gentle input which our organisms need. Reich seldom used the word 'trauma', but the *concept* of chronic traumatisation is central to his work, and to ours. 'Armouring' is one way to describe some of its effects.

ARMOURING AND ILLNESS

We've used the word 'healthy' once or twice to describe the state of natural, unarmoured openness, which can tend to make Reichian therapy sound like a medical technique. It isn't (although Reich fell into this trap at times): unlike medical treatment, there is no fixed intended outcome, just a general aim of greater freedom and spaciousness. But it is also the case that being armoured is a precondition for being ill in the medical sense. When energy can't flow freely through the body, we get areas that are over-charged, where energy 'sticks' and stagnates, and other areas that are undercharged, where energy can't get to at all. Over time, this sets up a chronic imbalance in the tissues and organs, which allows infection or functional disorder to take hold.

The sort of ailment which results is by no means random: our illnesses express, in vivid dumb show, the issues around which we tense and close off. To pick some trivial examples, often people who have a cough are suppressing anger – if you pretend to cough, and then exaggerate it, you will find yourself roaring. Similarly, colds often have to do with unexpressed grief – the tears have to find some way out.

This is a tremendous over-simplification: every illness is the expression of a complex and long-standing set of issues, involving interpersonal, social, psychological and biological factors. But we do see physical symptoms as the bodymind's attempt to resolve conflict, to break free from the constraints of the armouring. In Chapter 4 we shall look in more detail at the relationship between specific illnesses and specific forms of armouring.

Exercise 4
Think of some illness you have currently or have had in the past. Pick one of its symptoms, and imagine producing that symptom deliberately, as a mime or dumb show, a way of telling people something about how you are feeling. What would you be telling them?

3

Surrender

> Disappointment is a good sign of basic intelligence. It cannot be compared to anything else: it is so sharp, precise, obvious and direct ... Once we open ourselves, then we land on what is.
>
> Chögyam Trungpa, *Cutting Through Spiritual Materialism*

In the last chapter we saw that what Freud (or his translators) called the Ego can be understood as 'the grip we get on ourselves', the self-image which knits together bodily impulses and sensations into a whole. In practice we do this by rejecting a whole crowd of impulses as 'not *really* me', thus making these feelings unconscious. This is what happens mentally; the bodily parallel is that we take on a pattern of chronic tension which is constantly preventing certain movements and expressions – they 'just don't feel natural'. The 'Spastic I', with its terror of letting go, is identical with the spastic musculature, *unable* to let go because the holding on isn't even conscious.

But the 'I' doesn't *have* to be like this – or we would be in a real mess. It is possible to have a sense of self that is relaxed, flexible, open to change and spontaneity, able to surrender to our own impulses and to the reality of the world around us.

Any sort of self-awareness and intention is going to carry muscle *tone* – the difference between a limp, flaccid arm, and one which is relaxed but energised and ready for action. However, if we keep ourselves *permanently* ready for action, we tend to lose the capacity to relax; this is what is called a chronic anxiety state, or stress. It produces a rigid, inflexible body, and an 'I' to match. Or alternatively, we can give up, go limp, and let go of muscle tone completely – which is no more relaxed than the rigid option.

So what makes possible a relaxed 'I', a subtle, flexible, pulsating bodymind? The keyword is 'surrender': not to anyone or anything *else*, but to *ourselves*.

For some people the idea of surrender to ourselves, to our own feelings, will make immediate sense. For others it needs more explanation: it involves one of the central ways in which therapy is different from everyday ways of being in our society – one of therapy's *radical* aspects.

If it's raining outside, we don't generally say – or not at least without conscious childishness – 'But it *mustn't* rain any more, it's been raining all day and I don't *want* it to!' However, people constantly take this sort of attitude towards their emotions: 'I can't go on crying like this'; 'I've no right to feel so angry'; 'I must stop being frightened'.

We suggest that your feelings are like the weather: there's no sense in arguing with them.

If I am in a state of sorrow, for instance, then it makes no difference how 'good' or 'bad' the reasons are. The sorrow is *there*, a unitary bodymind state, woven of ideas, emotions, physiological changes, energy flows. I can't expunge it by an act of will. All I can do is stop myself *expressing* it, and perhaps blank out my consciousness of it. What this ensures is that *my sorrow will continue* – forever, quite possibly; locked up in the muscles I've tensed to stop myself sobbing and weeping; locked up in my unconscious mind. It won't simply go away.

The paradox is that feelings change through and in their expression. It's by opening to my sorrow, or anger, or fear, or joy, by truly accepting that this is, for now, my reality, that I am able to move beyond it. To complete themselves, feelings generally have to pass through consciousness and out again: it seems to be the only exit.

We experience this extraordinary miracle over and over again: just by surrendering to our feelings, we see them change. The trap that seemed inescapable, the wound that seemed unhealable, the dilemma that seemed insoluble – suddenly they are different – smaller, softer and more malleable, because our whole bodymind is softer and more flexible in its approach to the world.

Surrendering to our feelings is not about giving in to difficulties, but about liberating our energies to confront them in whatever way is appropriate. To face the world we need to face ourselves, as we are rather than as we would like to be. Neither is this to say that we should switch off our intelligence. We have to acknowledge sometimes that our emotional reaction is over the top, irrational, that we are responding to old memories and not to present facts. But this acknowledgement provides the context in which we can effectively let go *to* the feelings and thus let go *of* them – knowing them for what they are.

Emotions *always* have a rational basis. Fear is the bodymind's shrinking away from real threat; anger is its mobilisation, a flamethrower to blast away whatever blocks our creative expression. Often, though, this rational basis is in the past not the present: we are responding in ways that were appropriate for vulnerable children, but are no longer appropriate for adults with a potential for strong and independent action.

> **Exercise 5**
> Bring to mind some feeling that you have about another person, and which you feel is wrong, unreasonable and unfair. Just for a minute, let go of those judgements and ask yourself what is the grain of truth in your feeling. See whether you can let yourself just have it, without holding back or suppressing. Imagine that the other person might be able to receive your feeling without being hurt and defensive, and take in that you were upset with them. How does your body respond to all this?

It is often helpful to have a safe space in which we can express our feelings away from the people who may have sparked them off: for instance, a therapy session where we can beat up a cushion rather than our lover. At other times, though, the appropriate form of discharge is in real life action, by getting angry with whoever is oppressing us and making them stop.

We can use our heads, and other people's, to work out which sort of situation is which, to disentangle the mixture of past and present which is usually involved. We can deal with the Jobcentre people much more effectively if we aren't seeing them as our mother, giving or withholding vital nourishment; or with our boss if we aren't seeing them as an authoritarian father. Often it's good to try hitting the cushion first, and see what rational here-and-now core of feeling is left afterwards. And of course other options, like tearing up paper, or stamping our feet, or simply pretending (out loud) to tell the person off, may be more helpful in particular situations.

The key point is that emotions are e-motions, movements *out*, their natural function is precisely to clear what stops us moving on. Feelings are value-neutral, neither good nor bad, simply *there*. It's not our feelings that cause us trouble, but our feelings *about* feelings, our shame, embarrassment, denial – our resistance.

'Resistance' is a word for all the ways in which people seek to avoid their own movement, their own living process. And one paradoxical form that resistance can take is to beat ourselves up about our own resistance! 'Oh God, I'm so blocked. Why can't I let go, why can't I change?' It is important to see that resistance in therapy is like resistance in politics – it originates in *fighting oppression*.

If a child finds its feelings invalidated by the adult world in the ways we discussed in the last chapter, this is oppression of a very powerful kind. It's a life-threatening experience, and the child responds like a resistance movement in an occupied country – by going underground. We have all built up defences against outside threat and inside emotion for the best possible reasons, and in the best possible way. So let's congratulate ourselves, and respect our resistance as we might respect a guerrilla leader from some past war of liberation. The only trouble is that the guerrilla leader may have got stuck in a posture that actually obstructs the liberation for which she was fighting!

If we think a little more about the guerrilla war metaphor, we can see that resistance takes many forms. Guerrillas tend to avoid direct confrontation. Among the techniques they use are sabotage, going on strike, using decoys, changing the traffic signs, pretending ignorance, taking hostages .... All of these have parallels in the ways that we learn to resist internally. Therapy is one way of investigating this sort of situation. Almost certainly our circumstances will have changed since childhood, and it would probably make sense to revise some of our past decisions, let go of some of our resistance, let go of some of the limitations we have placed on our self-expression.

What we are really talking about is surrender to *reality*: the reality of our own feelings, and of the interactions which spark them off; the reality of the past, and of the present; the reality of our body's need for breath, for pleasure, for rest, for activity. Because the reality which confronts us is constantly changing, we need to be very flexible in order to deal with it: we need to be secure enough to face the bad along with the good, rather than run away into fantasy. That security and flexibility are rooted in a sense of *belonging*, being part of the universe, being fed by it in a constant pulsating exchange of energies: a sense that is part of our natural birthright, and is inherent in full free breathing.

SEX AND SURRENDER

To stay soft and open, we need the capacity to discharge tension that builds up in us through the stresses of living. Free breathing helps to minimise this build-up – we let go of tension with each outbreath. But the 'I' needs periodically to let go completely, to 'melt' as the armoured muscles melt, to relinquish control and allow the spontaneous rhythms of the organism to emerge. A natural, innate, powerful way of doing this is through lovemaking and orgasm: insofar as we can surrender to our own body, its pleasure washes us free of the tensions and blockings that have built up. The movements of orgasmic release are wavelike, pulsating, an involuntary contraction and relaxation of the whole body that transcends consciousness.

So can we all get healthy or stay healthy by making love? If only it was that simple. For a few people it is, or nearly so. It's one of those catch-22 situations: the more soft and open you are already, the easier it is to stay so. The way our body seeks to move in orgasm is totally different in nature from the controlled, circumspect movements of the armoured bodymind. The 'Spastic I' perceives involuntary movement – in a sense, quite rightly – as a dreadful threat to its survival. It panics, and clamps down even harder – perhaps tries to take control of the orgasmic movements, to 'let go on purpose'. For most of us, making love creates tension at the same time as releasing it.

Orgasmic surrender cannot really be separated from surrender to life and spontaneity in general, surrender to our selves. The way we relate to sexual excitement matches the way we relate to other sorts of stimulus: the way we live our lives. So the work that we do is not 'sex therapy'; but neither do we seek to disguise the central role of sexuality in life, and of orgasm as a form of discharge. We are also well aware that much of people's unconscious anxiety and tension has a specifically sexual content.

Orgasm in the sense of surrender to the involuntary is something rather different from simple mechanical spasm or heavy breathing. Many people influenced by Reich's ideas have made something of a fetish out of the 'Total Orgasm', treating it as a specific goal, something you either 'get' or 'don't get'. This is unrealistic, and very much at odds with Reich's central point about letting go and saying yes to our pleasure wherever it takes us. (Reich himself was not able to follow through consistently with his own best insights.) Sexual release is a primary form of discharge, a way to stay soft and sweet. But it can be directly worked for and learnt only in limited ways: it is above all a function of our overall openness and capacity to handle pleasure and excitement.

So our therapy doesn't simply work on sexuality as such, or on tension in the pelvic area alone. It seeks to encourage an overall loosening of the armour, a release of anxiety which will make it possible to give in to our own impulse for genital pleasure. Breathing is an accessible yardstick of openness and spontaneity, and Reich noticed that when a person is relaxed and breathing freely and fully, the movement of her body is similar, in a gentle and uncharged way, to the movement of orgasm. As we breathe out, lying on our backs, the pelvic rocks *forward* and *up*, while at the same time our throat comes forward as if to meet our pelvis. Our head and shoulders fall back and open in a vulnerable gesture of surrender. This is identical for men and women.

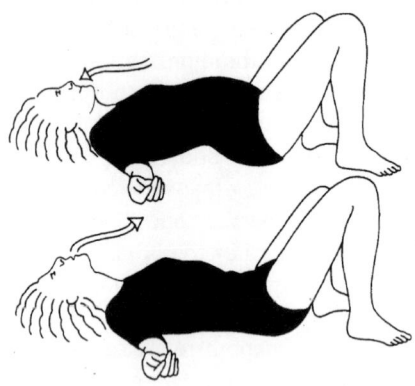

So now you can go off and practise free breathing! This won't do you any harm, but it is unlikely to do you much good either. We can't practise the spontaneous or will the involuntary; what is crucial is the feeling-tone of the movement, rather than its mechanical 'correctness'. Reich called this full, free breath the 'orgasm reflex'; by definition, a reflex is something which bypasses conscious control.

Full, free breathing is not a state, but a direction: we can always breathe more or less than we are doing at the moment. Exploring what happens as we try to alter or increase our breath – or rather, to stop holding it back and distorting it – is a direct route to the heart of therapy, involving us in a long-term project of melting armour in all parts of our body, all aspects of our character. When we find ourselves, for a while, breathing very freely, we experience all sorts of strange and pleasurable sensations in our bodyminds, an opportunity to directly perceive the flow of life energy in ourselves, which Reich called 'streaming'.

The flow of Orgone is immediately experienced as pleasure; its blocking as unpleasure.

But pleasure, for most people, is very often bound up with anxiety. It makes the 'Spastic I' feel that it is losing its identity; it brings back bodymind memories of childhood situations where our pleasure was frustrated, together with the associated feelings of grief, fear and rage. If our first reaction to pleasure beyond a certain limit is *no* rather than *yes*, then our wires need uncrossing. We need to unpeel, layer by layer, the different negative feelings that have come to overlay our innately joyful, playful response to energy flow.

But it's plain too that making love isn't *vital* to being in a good state. There are many people, for example, who are celibate but who use meditation or other bodymind disciplines to keep themselves soft and clear. It's also *very* plain – as Reich was well aware – that sexual activity as such is no measure of health or pleasure – frantic fucking can be precisely an avoidance of surrender.

So if you don't seek orgasmic surrender, perhaps the best question is 'Why not?' Some reasons are better than others. A long-term relationship may go through effectively 'asexual' phases, and yet both partners feel it would be destructive to look for sexual satisfaction elsewhere.

Also, sex and sexuality in our culture carry a tremendous weight of *political* meanings which make it hard to simply follow our feelings: our feelings may be contradictory. Above all, the role of patriarchal power in our society has a profound effect on both heterosexual and homosexual love. We'll come back to these matters in Chapters 6 and 9; for now, we just want to say that because of this political charge, sexual surrender becomes even more frightening. Surrender to our own feelings is not easily separated from surrender to someone else, or to a particular sexual ideology. It can be difficult to disentangle saying 'yes' to our bodies from saying 'yes' to patriarchy, because in a sense we may experience our bodies as colonised and imperialised by society's models of sexuality, power and pleasure.

The way forward through this jungle, hard though it is, is surely to stay with exactly what comes up for us when we try to let go, breathe, and feel our bodymind. If we can accept and own our sensations and emotions, without judgement or denial, then we can eventually find the way through to our truth, a truth based on far more solid foundations than any intellectual model. This means being able to face the pain and fear of our original childhood confrontation with sexual roles and rules.

In the next chapter, we shall look at the way we tighten up each area of our body, each segment of armouring, against surrender to feeling, to pleasure, and to reality.

4

The Segments

> The segmental arrangement of the muscular armour represents the worm in man.
>
> Wilhelm Reich, *Character Analysis*

Now let us look at how armouring works in practice: where the different 'segments' are located, the sorts of emotions that tend to be stuck unexpressed and unexperienced in the tense muscles of each body area, and the sorts of physical symptoms that tend to accompany these tensions.

What follows is necessarily simplified. Although the seven segments can be a tremendously useful way of seeing patterns of holding, they are only a tool – only one way of seeing things. As we go through the segments, we will be constantly pointing out interconnections between them and other, equally valid, ways of understanding our bodies. The segments are to a large extent an artificial system; but this can be seen as reflecting the artificial bodymind process of self-armouring. Hence the illustration of the segments shows a highly 'artificial' looking figure, someone from the Middle Ages or science fiction!

One thing to get clear at the start is that people usually don't know about their own armouring. After all, the whole purpose of the muscle tension is to protect us from consciously realising our feelings and needs. It also tends to make us unaware of the tension itself, which through long familiarity feels 'normal', in the same sort of way that water seems tasteless because we have its taste permanently in our mouths. In a sense the purpose of Reichian therapy is to help people become fully aware of their own muscular tension, which makes it possible (though not necessarily easy) for the muscles to relax. At this point the feelings and images which re-enter our awareness may come as quite a shock.

Another thing to bear in mind is that instead of being charged up with intense held feeling, a segment can in effect be 'emptied' of charge, made limp and without energy, because the person is using an alternative self-control strategy: tense muscles around the area are keeping energy and feelings *out*. Also, there is more than one layer of musculature in any given area of our body; we may be relaxed at one level, tight at another. All of this should become clearer as we go on.

The seven segments, as shown in the illustration, can be identified by the main feature of each area – the eyes; the jaw; the throat; the heart; the waist; the belly; and the pelvis and legs. We shall look at each in turn, working down the body in the direction that an embryo grows in the womb, the direction that our bodywork tends to move, from crown to base. Take this chapter slowly, spending some time with each segment and fully noticing your own reactions. As we said in the last chapter, reading about these matters can be very stirring.

The segments of armouring

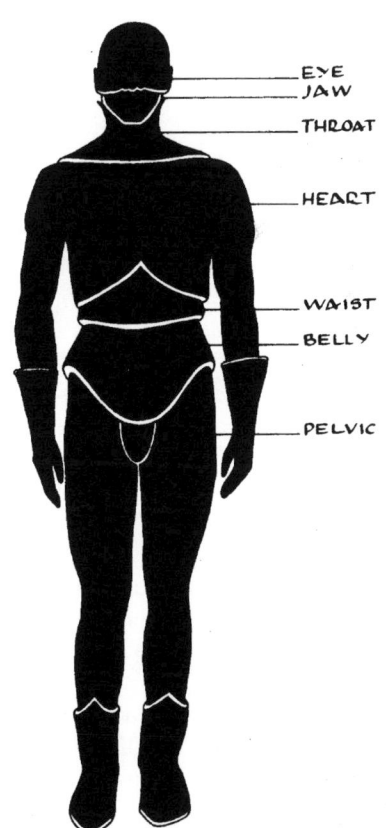

THE EYE SEGMENT ('OCULAR')

The first and uppermost segment includes the scalp, forehead, eyes, cheeks, ears, and the base of the skull. It is an area of intense charge, containing as it does two crucial 'windows' on the world, our organs of sight and hearing. Whether because of this, or because of the location of the brain, most people mentally place their 'I' in this segment; this is where we watch the world from, where we think, where we imagine that we press the buttons and move the levers to work our body.

Eye segment: showing the muscles around the eye

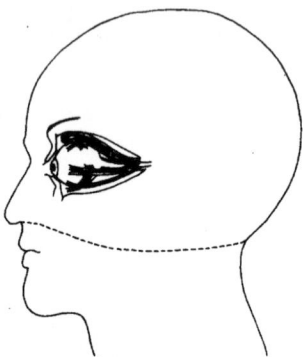

Such notions and experiences are themselves a product of armouring. They show the extent of cut-offness from our heart, guts and sex. The mind is a bodymind – not a headmind – however 'natural' it may seem to be 'in our heads'. The neuroscientist Antonio Damasio argues that our sense of self is essentially a sense of our body, and that *our whole body thinks*, not just our head.

One very common effect of working to melt the armour is that people's centre of awareness shifts downwards, into the 'heartlands' of the body. We begin to experience our heads, weirdly at first, as just another limb like our arms or legs. We start to realise how stiffly we have been holding our head, so as to stay 'in' it; and how tension in and around our eyes represents the need to 'hold ourselves up' through seeing, rather than through the support of our legs and feet – desperately gripping on to the world with our eyes, in the same sort of way that when we were learning to stand we kept ourselves erect by gripping on with our hands.

As well as being a vital channel for information and contact, eyes and ears have also been a source of *threat* in our lives. Scary and existence-threatening energy has invaded us through our sight and hearing – the coldness or resentment in the look of adults who should be caring for us, for example, the anger, pain or indifference in their voices. Most of us came into the world in the agonising glare of hospital lights, the cacophony of hospital noises; later, we may have tried to minimise dangerous excitement by 'not looking', 'not seeing' stirring images, 'not hearing' the confusing sounds of our parents arguing or making love.

So very often the eyes and ears are in a permanent state of blocking, which says 'I won't see – won't hear – won't understand'. Muscles inside and around the eye sockets and at the base of the skull are in constant tension, stopping us from really focusing on the world around us, from opening up to reality.

> **Exercise 6**
>
> Try an experiment yourself: sit upright, and turn your head as far as it will comfortably go to one side. When it reaches a stopping point let your eyes carry on round until they too reach their comfortable limit – no need to strain; then bring the eyes very slowly back round until, as they face forward again in the head, they 'pick up' the head and both continue moving back round to the front of the body. The illustration should make this clear. The point is that the eyes should move continuously, without jumping, so they 'sweep' the field of vision, carrying the head along with them. Keep breathing while you do it!

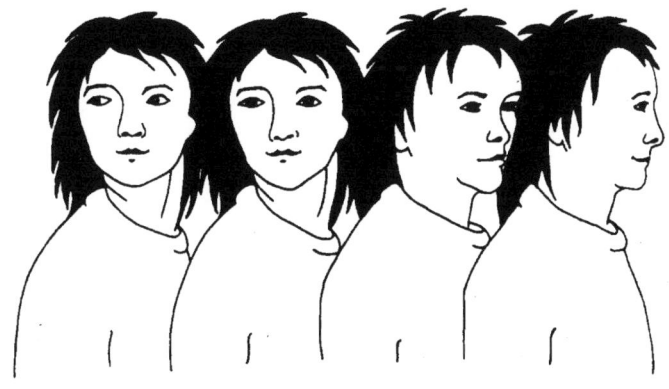

Most people find this exercise very difficult – to let their eyes move slowly and continuously rather than jumping forward in spurts, impatient to see 'what's next'. This impatience has a quality of fear in it, and repeating the experiment a few times to each side can make us conscious of a great deal of anxiety about seeing, *really seeing*, the world around us. We tend to filter reality through a screen of prior judgement so as to protect ourselves from dangerous excitement or pain, and this anxiety is bound into tense muscles around the eyes.

A similar process happens with the ears, and with our thinking processes. The words we use about thinking embody these connections: 'I see what you mean', 'I don't like the sound of that'. In French, *'entendu'* means both 'heard' and 'understood'.

The core of the armouring is actually *inside* the head, in the small muscles that move our eyes, and in the muscles behind our ears and at the base of the skull, some of which are reflexly coordinated with subtle eye movements. Blocking in all these areas can give a hard, blank, superficial expression to the eyes, or a cloudy 'absent look' – both masking deep fear. Shortsightedness, longsightedness, deafness, etc., are very much bound up with armouring of the eye segment, and the same goes for inability to smell – a very powerful and fundamental sense linking us with our animal heritage.

Repression of contact with the world through eyes, ears and thinking covers up a deeper *neediness*. Eye contact which is loving and supportive gives us a fundamental anchoring in the world: it says 'you exist, I see you'. When the channels are open, the heart speaks through the eyes, and comforting sounds and smells can give an almost equally deep reassurance. If this sort of validation is missing in very early childhood, then someone's ability to make proper contact through the eye segment can be profoundly injured. They tend to 'go away in the eyes' and in their thinking: closeness can be experienced as invasive, threatening – only in isolation are they safe. Similarly they may develop ideas which are bizarrely isolated from how most people see the world.

With less extreme damage, the urge for contact may simply take a diversion, and express itself in a way which is distorted and therefore less threatening: as with people whose life is organised around a *need to see* – voyeurs, intellectuals, detectives, journalists – and therapists! Which is a good moment to stress that reaching out with eyes, ears and mind is a healthy, creative process – unless it coincides with a block to making deep emotional contact.

As well as being windows, the eyes are doors: they are a channel for emotional expression. *All* feelings, to be fully released, need to come out through the eyes. Besides the obvious example of crying, the eyes must release fear, anger, joy, and so on in appropriate ways in order to stay soft and open. Different people tend to be able to show different feelings through their eyes, and to block other ones; and these tendencies can often be seen in the way we hold the muscles of this segment.

> **Exercise 7**
>
> Look in a mirror, and raise your eyebrows as far as you possibly can. What does this look like? What emotion does it convey? Now screw your eyes up tight, lower the brow: see what the apparent emotion is now. Keep breathing, and move as fast as you can between these two positions, several times; how does this make you feel? Is it easy for you to do? Is one position harder than the other? Relax into your normal eye position for a moment, let yourself breathe, and see how you look in the mirror and how you feel inside.

As we hope you will agree, the wide-open eyes show an expression of *fear*; and if you kept breathing in this position, you may even have felt some of this fear. People who habitually keep their eyes like this are generally unaware of it; getting them to exaggerate, or conversely to screw their eyes up tight, can make them suddenly aware of the extreme tension there, and of the underlying fear and sadness. It's a position which helps one cope with being seen, and is common in politicians and others in the public view, but also in people who have had very frightening visual experiences in childhood.

Screwed-up eyes may convey several different emotions: anger, desperation to see, anxiety. Notice whether your cheek muscles also screw up tight, turning your face into a mask. When people habitually use their faces in this way, it's as if their eyes have retreated into their head – 'I can see out, but you can't see in'. Flat, stiff, heavy cheeks, on the other hand, are often holding tremendous grief and unshed tears.

Another emotion often held in the eye segment is *worry:* the wrinkled brow and fixed gaze of compulsive thinking. It doesn't matter what the person is thinking about *now* – it could be absolutely anything – but originally they will have taken refuge in thinking as an escape route from intolerable childhood pressures, for example, trying to work out how to satisfy contradictory demands from mother and father.

The 'ivory tower intellectual' is demonstrating a similar, perhaps more successful, form of escape: the skull is a literal ivory tower, high and dry above the scary and confusing world of the body. Intellectuals who try to ignore body and emotions have concentrated on the genuine erotic pleasure of thought to the exclusion of most other things.

Thinking is a real, healthy pleasure, but surely only in harmony with other functions, not in isolation from them. Often there is considerable panic bound up in this stance – about sexual feelings, and also about bodily assertiveness and rage. The opposite form of defence is found in people who fog up their own thinking processes as a protection against painful realities, *making* themselves stupid and incompetent, and giving their eyes either a dull smug look ('It's no good talking to me'), or a peering vagueness.

These are some examples to stimulate your own observation of what people do with their eyes. The eye segment will be involved in suppressing any and all feelings; but the fundamental blockings here are of very *young* emotions and experiences, our primal interactions with the world, starting at birth or earlier. Through the crown of our heads and the space between and above our eyes, we are linked to sky and cosmos, to webs of subtle energy, to something much bigger than our individual self. Pain and danger may make us close these channels down, or may make us retreat into a 'spirituality' which is ungrounded in the reality of our bodily life.

Apart from defects of vision and hearing, the most obvious physical symptom connected with eye segment armouring is chronic headaches, stemming from tense muscles at the base of the skull and around the eyes (which may themselves come from tension at more distant points). We believe as well that specific ailments like sties, conjunctivitis, sinusitis and so on can be linked with eye segment armouring; often they occur when a specific feeling is being held back about some life situation, and in particular when someone is not allowing themselves to cry.

JAW AND MOUTH SEGMENT ('ORAL')

Just as all emotions need to be expressed through the eyes to complete themselves, so they also need to be expressed in *sound* – sobbing, yelling, sighing, screaming, laughing. The mouth and jaw are clearly a key part of the vocalising process: when armoured they form a 'lid' to the expressive channel, either closing the voice off entirely or else deadening and flattening it. Sound may emerge mechanically, but it lacks meaning and vibrancy as long as the jaw is tight. We can learn to recognise the dead, droning or quacking tone of an armoured jaw; we all know to avoid someone who sounds like a bore.

The Segments   35

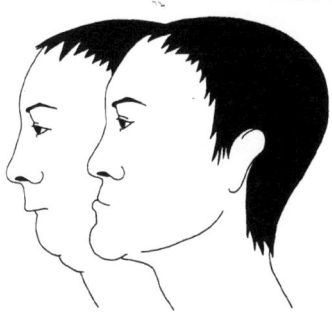

An underlying fear of expressing one particular emotion can set up a block that affects *all* expression. With the jaw, there is very often some held back *anger*: a desire to growl, roar and bite which, when suppressed, can create a fixed unreal grin of underlying hatred. This held back rage – the 'Wolfman' in all of us – is simply frustrated love and wanting, a softness that has turned hard in self-protection. Every time a child is stopped from saying what she wants, every time she is force-fed with food she doesn't want, the anger builds up. And usually, the anger itself is prevented from expression by adult sanctions – like a hand held over the mouth, a hand we want to bite and tear.

To many people, the idea that we have such feelings seems dreadful and unacceptable. It is often those who on the surface are mildest and gentlest who are holding the most rage in their jaws. But real sweetness and melting is only possible once the hate is discharged. Often people need to gag and cough to release their 'swallowed' feelings (see also the section below on the throat segment).

Anger in the jaw is thus very closely related to defiance and stubbornness: 'I won't let you see my hurt'. Many of us as children felt that showing our anger represented defeat and punishment. We might be laughed at, so we learnt to tighten our mouth and push our chin forward in a habitual gesture of silent resistance. Or we started to pull our chin *back* in an expression which says 'I'm harmless': people with retracted chins are usually over-positive and determinedly cheerful whatever their true circumstances.

**Jaw segment:
showing the masseter and temporalis muscles**

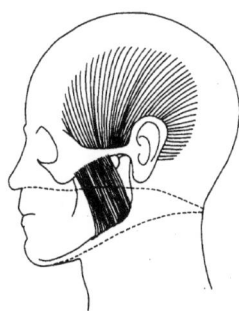

> **Exercise 8**
> You can experiment in front of the mirror, pushing your chin forward and pulling it back as far as possible – while still breathing. How do these positions make you feel? What effect do they have on the rest of your face, if any? Does one feel easier or more natural than the other? Move between them a few times, then let your jaw relax and see how it looks and feels.
>
> And while you're at it, do what a child does when trying to hold back tears: tighten your chin muscles up, clamping your lips together.

This 'stiff lower lip' is an expression we can all recognise in children, and in very many adults who keep these muscles permanently stiff, holding back a deep and by now unconscious sadness. This may be combined with a tension *under* the jaw, an area linked with the tongue muscles, which should be soft and supple but in adults seldom is. The sound held in this region is the angry yell of a baby whose needs are not being recognised.

> **Exercise 9**
>
> The simplest way to check out the armouring of your jaw segment is to look in the mirror, raise your chin slightly, and let your mouth drop open. Don't force it, but just see how far it falls under its own weight. If your jaw is free, then the 'hinge' muscles in front of the ears will let it drop wide open – enough, say, to insert three fingers sideways on between your upper and lower teeth; but more likely, there will be one or another sort of holding that keeps your mouth half closed. Breathing freely with your jaw dropped like this could put you in touch with the specific emotions and tensions around your jaw.

As with the eyes, under the hard blocking in the jaw are soft feelings of need. Naturally enough, these are very much bound up with feeding, and the baby's pleasure in sucking: any disturbance in this phase of life will be reflected later in jaw armouring – especially anger and disappointment about not being fed when hungry, harsh or premature weaning, or a general lack of warm contact in the feeding relationship.

It is widely accepted that we pick up many of our mother's emotions through her milk: its hormone balance varies with her state of being. And more generally, both breast- and bottle-fed babies are highly sensitive to the feeling-connection with their mother or any nurturing adult: her involvement or preoccupation, her happiness or sadness. Our reactions to this, our feelings of not getting what we need from her, will lodge among other places in the jaw segment.

The muscles which move our jaw link in to the base of the skull, which is thus a point of connection between eye and jaw segments: a crucial body area which often collects a good deal of tension, and sometimes has to deal with real contradictions between the two segments: a person's face may be split in two, so that the eyes and mouth express quite different emotions, for example happiness in the mouth and fear in the eyes.

Migraine headaches have been linked with tension in the jaw, causing a displaced bite which transmits up into the head. Tooth and gum problems of all kinds are related to suppressed emotions and the resulting tension; in particular we have noticed a relationship between tooth abscesses and the need to express hidden anger. Coughs and colds can be part of a suppressive or releasing process in this area.

THROAT AND NECK SEGMENT ('CERVICAL')

In each segment it is possible and often helpful to distinguish a soft, inside, 'Yin' aspect (often in the front) and a hard, outside, 'Yang' aspect. For the jaw this is represented in the difference between the sucking, melting impulses of the tongue and palate, and the assertive biting and growling of the teeth and chin. With this segment the difference is particularly clear between the softness of the throat and the hardness of the neck.

Neck/throat segment: showing the sternocleidomastoid muscle

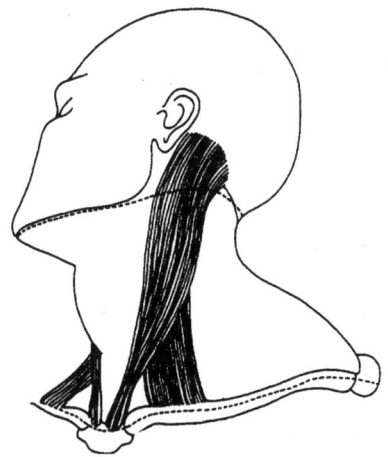

Much of the expressive energy that develops in our torso has to work its way up through the narrow channel of the throat in order to emerge through the mouth and eyes. It's not surprising that this passage easily becomes jammed up, and the word anxiety itself comes from the Latin *angustus*, which means 'narrow'. The choking, strangling, 'can't get through' feeling of jammed up energy can set up tremendous anxiety in the throat area, sensations which we probably associate unconsciously with birth – with being stuck, half-suffocated, in another narrow passage, perhaps even with the cord around our neck, certainly with our throat full of mucus. In bodywork therapy a huge amount of coughing is sometimes necessary to 'clear the throat', both energetically and emotionally. Mucus has a strange capacity to create itself, as it seems, out of nowhere, as a representation or embodiment of held feelings.

In fact, one of the most powerful and therapeutic tools can be to help someone to retch and gag, while breathing and letting the sound come. All the 'swallowing down' of feelings that we've been doing for a lifetime is turned round; the energy starts to move up and out, and we experience it directly as a melting and softening of throat, jaw and eyes all at once. There is also a lot of fear released – many people hate gagging and are scarcely ever sick, mainly because they unconsciously feel they must keep their feelings down at all costs. When someone becomes secure and strong enough to let herself retch, the effect can be astonishingly liberating. On the other hand, there are people who retch and gag very easily, and often, as a way of avoiding having to take in and digest feelings. Anything, including expressiveness, can be used as a defence!

The fear held in the throat seems to have a different quality from that of the eye segment. The eyes are afraid of invasion and dissolution on what we can call an 'existential' level, while the throat often seems to hold a fear of real bodily death rather than ego annihilation. It's as if our birth process is also our introduction to the reality of death – and the throat is a place where this death-fear roosts in us. Then, later on, it attracts to itself our fear of our own murderous impulses. We strangle ourselves on our own hatred as the urge to hit and hurt and tear, which develops in our hands if our love and pleasure are frustrated, gets pulled back up our arms and jammed into the muscles round the base of our throat. We turn our anger on ourselves, and strangle ourselves rather than someone else.

This is a complicated and important sequence, an excellent example of how armouring forms, and it's worth going over it again to help make the process clear. Notice, to begin with, that from our viewpoint the anger and aggression are not *primary* (as they would be for some other therapies): human nature does not involve wanting to hurt people, but wanting to love and be loved, to make warm contact. It is when this warmth is rejected that anger – quite appropriately – comes, but children's fear of adult violence then often intervenes to block any direct 'hot' expression of anger. The *outward* movement, first of love and pleasure then of rage, becomes an *inward* retreat, which tends to stick at the base of the throat. Warmth turns to cold, and freezes our muscles.

Thus, because we can't vent frustration, we block off our search for love as well. Hands can't reach out for contact, throats can't open in a giving, surrendering way as they want to do. Often, before they can have soft feelings in their throat, people need to act out a state very like the stereotype fairytale witch with her strangled cackle, claw-like hands and spiteful hate, which very accurately portray a throat block!

Although hands and arms connect mainly with the heart segment, we have just seen that they also relate strongly to the throat. We can see too how the throat links in strongly with the mouth and jaw: sucking and voice both involve both segments. One could say that the neck, in contrast, links via the base of the skull to the eyes. The neck has the job of supporting the head, and the attitude that the eye segment takes towards the world will very much affect and be affected by how the neck operates.

If the eyes are holding on desperately, then the neck will tend to be correspondingly rigid and inflexible – a proud, 'stiff-necked' attitude may manifest, covering up deeper fear. The more that someone is stuck in their head as opposed to inhabiting the whole body, the more tension will be found in their neck – it has to stop the head from failing off, floating up, or being flooded with body-feelings. The neck may be stretched out nervously into the world, or protectively scrunched up into the shoulders like a turtle.

So the combination of eye-linked neck and jaw-linked throat can produce all sorts of different postures in this segment. Two very important muscles are the big sternocleidomastoids, which run on either side from the base of the skull just behind the ears, round the side of the neck, down to the front of the breastbone holding the entire segment together. You may notice that when you are tired and tense these muscles become painful. Many headaches originate here and slowly work their way up into our heads as we try to force ourselves to feel all right by stiffening the posture of our head and neck.

Often there is a tendency in people to pull the head back, scrunching up the base of the skull as if to say 'I'm undefeated, I won't bow down', but at the same time retreating from facing the world in front of them. In fact this posture is often associated with shortsightedness; longsightedness being associated with pushing the head forward.

Many of us are afraid to let our necks go fully, and (as the Alexander Technique emphasises) holding on here can be the central cause of tension and contraction patterns throughout the body.

> **Exercise 10**
> You can explore the state of your neck by lying on your back with your head on something soft, and turning it from side to side as rapidly as possible. Don't hold your breath. If you can, let your head flop completely from side to side – and leave your shoulders flat on the floor, just moving head and neck. Does this make you sick and dizzy? If so, it's an indication of tension. Also, try lifting your head and bringing it down strongly onto a pillow. Repeat several times; keep breathing, and again, don't use your shoulders. What does this feel like? If possible, get a friend to help by putting their hands round and under your head, and lifting it gently, moving it from side to side and up and down. Can you let them control the movement, or do you involuntarily help them with your own muscles? Do you have a similar need to stay in charge in your life?

HEART SEGMENT ('THORACIC')

The chest, shoulders and upper back, arms and hands, between them make up the heart segment which must be open for us to express 'big' feelings, strong, expansive emotions, coming out in full resonant voice and powerful gestures. For most of us the heart is to a greater or lesser extent closed off, injuring our capacity for deep feeling and deep contact; because, consciously or unconsciously, it feels bruised, or broken, or frozen, or imprisoned, or hiding.

Chögyam Trungpa Rinpoche, a Tibetan teacher, tells us that true contact means taking on and owning a certain painfulness that goes with being open: 'The genuine heart of sadness comes from feeling that your nonexistent heart is full ... Real fearlessness is the product of tenderness. It comes from letting the world tickle your heart, your raw and beautiful heart. You are willing to open up, without resistance or shyness, and face the world. You are willing to share your heart with others.'

What accompanies this opening up on a bodily level is a melting of the muscular armour in chest and shoulders, so that we are able to breathe fully into our chest – and out again. There is very often some interruption to this full cycle of inbreath and outbreath. As we have seen, one person may hold her chest permanently half full of air, never breathing out, while another person may never really breathe *in*. Often there is a prolonged pause between breathing in and breathing out, or vice versa.

Heart segment: showing the movement of the ribs as we breathe

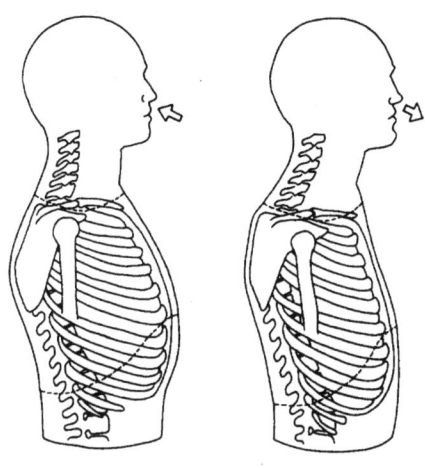

> **Exercise 11**
> If you return to the mirror, you may be able to see what these two opposite forms of holding mean. Breathe in as deeply as you can, and hold it: what does this look like? Now push all the air out of your lungs, and hold this position: what attitude to life are you portraying?

You may well find that with your chest held full, you look *afraid*. Gasping air is a reflex accompaniment to a frightening shock. A permanent gasp goes along with high tight shoulders, and often with clenched hands. These are all part of the same fear pattern, inscribed on the body by repeated frightening experiences in early life. The fear is often covered up with *defiance* – sticking out your chest to make yourself look big, clenching your fists to look aggressive – but there is a tension, and often a look of powerlessness, in the arms which reveals the underlying meaning. It's a common result of having an authoritarian father, and can often be seen in teenage gang members.

When you breathe out as far as possible, your chest now caves in and your shoulders slump down and forward: an image of *defeat*. People who are stuck in this sort of posture have generally given up. Through constant frustration, especially in early life, they have formed the idea that it is safest and least upsetting to have as little energy as possible in their bodies, so, as far as is compatible with staying alive, they've given up breathing in.

Which of these postures felt more natural and easy to you?

There are many styles of protecting our heart from the world. Some people's chests scarcely move at all as they breathe: if you press down gently on the breastbone, it feels like a solid plate of armour, or a thick layer of rubber. With others, the chest gives completely to the least pressure – there is no assertiveness at all, no sense of 'here I am'. Sometimes one feels afraid to press at all, there is such a sense of brittleness and fragility. Some people are 'pigeon-chested' or 'barrel-chested' – two different ways of sticking yourself out rigidly and ungivingly into the world, the first emphasising the upper and front chest, the second including the lower chest and sides; neither allowing the easy natural exchange of energies represented by the in and out of the breath. Everyone has their personal style of armouring.

Whatever else may be going on in a person, their shoulders are usually a reservoir of unexpressed rage. This rage, again, can be held in many different styles: high and tight, or pulled back to scrunch between the shoulder blades, or screwed up in the armpits. Generally it needs release via the arms, smashing your fists down on to a cushion, beating a mattress with your elbows (often necessary before energy can come down into the forearms and hands), scratching, tearing, pinching.

> **Exercise 12**
>
> You can find out how free your shoulders and arms are by moving them around: 'shrug' your shoulders in a circular movement from back to front, and then from front to back, working your elbows like a clucking chicken. Raise your arms slowly in front of you until they point right up in the air, then open them out at the sides to shoulder height. Remember to breathe while you do it! Are any of these movements difficult, physically or emotionally?

As the armouring of our chest and shoulders starts to dissolve, we come into our power. We sense ourselves as strong, real and formidable, without being aggressive or having anything to prove: a *soft* power, which asserts our need for contact yet is able to deal with hostility or coldness.

Crying is done with the chest as well as with the eyes and mouth. Sometimes people think they are crying when a few tears leak out, but without any deep sobbing that moves the heart and the whole being. The pain here may be much more profound and shaking, and along with this comes a much deeper release, a sense of inner cleansing and lightness on a different level from the effect of simple weeping.

The heart segment is the seat of much of our passion, our intensity and vibrancy. Only when we are willing and able to let our chest and shoulders move – *be* moved – with our breath, can we deeply and seriously engage with reality. We say 'seriously', but this doesn't imply anything solemn: among the emotions of the heart segment is robust, hearty laughter, often held back in 'ticklish' irritable muscles in the sides and under the arms. Tickling can be a remarkably effective bodywork technique; it helps to 'unstick' the ribs from each other, opening up the independent movement of the intercostal muscles.

Armouring in this segment has a negative effect on the functioning of the heart and lungs, predisposing these organs to disease. In particular we see a relationship between suppressed anger and bronchitis and chronic coughs; between deep fear and asthma; and between physical heart failure and 'heartbreak'.

WAIST SEGMENT ('DIAPHRAGMATIC')

As the illustration shows, the diaphragm is a big, dome-shaped muscle that runs right through the body at waist level, separating our upper and lower halves (with holes for the oesophagus, veins and arteries, etc.). Above it are the heart and lungs; below, the stomach, intestines, liver, pancreas, kidneys, and so on. The diaphragm attaches to our spine at the back, and to our bottom ribs, knitting our torso together and connecting also to our pelvis and hips.

It is primarily with the diaphragm that we breathe – or that at least is how our body is designed! If our diaphragm is mobile, then each inbreath starts with its contraction, so that the upward, dome-like bulge flattens out. This increases the space in the chest cavity, and the lungs automatically expand into the semi-vacuum, sucking in air. As the diaphragm relaxes, it bells out upward again, firmly pushing the air out of our lungs. Muscles in the ribcage, shoulders, etc., can *stop* us breathing by being too tight, but their role in *causing* us to breathe is secondary to that of this great, powerful sheet of muscle. Really, our chest muscles just have to get out of the way.

Waist segment: the diaphragm

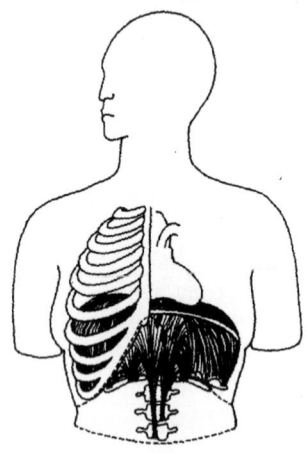

It is the diaphragm, therefore, which first tightens and freezes in unhappy babies, interrupting the spontaneous natural flow of breath. Thus this segment stores the intolerable primal terror that first made us cut off from our own energy; the sensation which, in a much diluted form, is familiar to most of us as 'butterflies in the tummy'.

A more intense version is often referred to as a 'sinking' feeling, a 'lurch' around the stomach, as if 'the bottom is dropping out'. This is a very accurate description of sudden movement in this boundary between our upper and lower internal world. The sinking feeling corresponds to a sense of falling *down into ourselves* – into the realm of 'gut feelings', emotions and sensations which are far less easily translatable into rational language than are those of our head and upper body.

Waist segment: how the diaphragm moves as we breathe

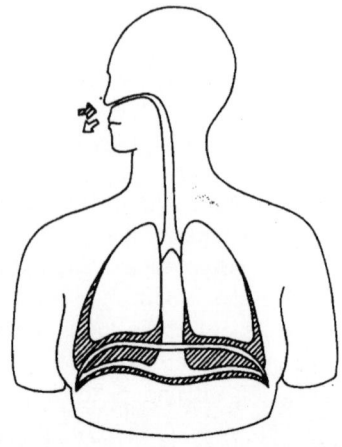

The more frozen the diaphragm, the more of an absolute division there will be between head and belly, between reason and instinct, between conscious and unconscious, 'heaven' and 'hell'. The diaphragm is turned into a 'floor'; and if the floor starts giving way as bodywork enables the diaphragm to move again, the experience can be deeply disturbing. People with tight diaphragms very often breathe with *either* chest *or* belly, or if both move, they can be quite unsynchronised, so that the belly may even be sinking as the chest rises and vice versa (though this is nothing to do with the yoga technique of 'paradoxical breathing').

> **Exercise 13**
>
> To get a sense of what is happening in your diaphragm, you can try rapidly panting from this area of your body. You need to breathe firmly in and equally firmly out again, rather than putting the emphasis on either one. Be aware that your sides and back around waist level should expand and contract as well – imagine a wide sash around your waist, stretching all round as you breathe in. Make the breathing continuous, breathing in again as soon as the outbreath is complete, and vice versa. You may find that a very few such breaths make you feel distinctly strange, with your head becoming dizzy and highly charged, and perhaps a slight nausea. This will pass off as soon as you stop – which you should obviously do when you get uncomfortable. This is a very early stage of panic, as you not only pass more breath-energy through your body, but also start to join up areas that you may habitually keep firmly separate.

The diaphragm often holds murderous rage as well as fear: a blind, total anger against the early repression that makes up our breathing armour. This anger can often be located in the sides and back of the waist segment, where the diaphragm anchors itself to bone – William West calls the side muscles here the 'spite muscles'. Lower-back tension, that classic twentieth-century problem, can often be related to a frozen diaphragm, and to conflicts between 'higher' and 'lower' needs and feelings – especially those involving the pelvis.

Thus a fundamental issue with the diaphragm is one of control. Problems in this area usually arise out of a struggle to 'control oneself' – that central, impossible instruction which our culture gives its children. Our nature as an organism demands spontaneity: only death is predictable, and predictability is death. The attempt to 'get a grip on ourselves' very much involves the diaphragm, one of the body's great core muscles, and seat of the involuntary/voluntary crossover at the centre of the breathing process. Only a few people can control their heartbeat, but all of us can control our breathing. In doing so habitually, we do ourselves great damage, yet the ability to be *aware* of our breath, to gently 'ride' its waves, is a deeply healing one. When the diaphragm is free and mobile, we are open to spontaneously arising material from 'the depths' – open to our *bellythink*.

There is a powerful reflex relationship between diaphragm and throat, such that armouring in one will be reflected in the other, and melting in one will likewise encourage melting in the other. If you listen to a 'catch' in a person's breath, you may be able to hear how it happens in both these places. Gagging and retching can be initiated in either the throat or the diaphragm, but they involve both. This is only one example of the complex system of reflex mirrorings in our body.

Tension in the waist will lay us open to *all* the stress-related ailments, since it disturbs our entire breathing pattern, with destructive effects on our metabolic processes. More specifically, it will tend to influence ailments like chronic nausea, ulcers (held-back frustration and rage), pancreatitis, gall and kidney stones and, as we have mentioned, lower-back pain.

BELLY SEGMENT ('ABDOMINAL')

The belly is a storehouse of unexpressed, unacknowledged feelings, images, ideas, desires and intentions – in effect a bodymind unconscious. The very word 'belly' is unspeakable to some people; they refer to it inaccurately as the 'stomach'! Here are the 'gut feelings', the instinctive self, and the more we are armoured higher up the body, the more these feelings are repressed. New material is being added all the time as we swallow down what we cannot say or do or feel.

The gurgling, bubbling belly is a place of water – the waters of life. Water needs to flow, or it becomes sour and stagnant and then this great subterranean sea turns into nothing but a huge septic tank. There is often much bitterness and stagnation down here in the body's underworld, expressed in toxicity, 'acid stomach', colitis and constipation – all of which reflect an inability to let go of waste and poison.

Our belly is vulnerable: the 'soft underbelly' of our stance towards the world. Insofar as we are insecure in the world, we tend to tense up our belly muscles, creating the macho, 'go on, hit me as hard as you like', image: or the flat, sucked-in little-girl tummy that women are encouraged to strive for. This impossibly flat, anorexic tummy is quite a recent invention. Renaissance and mediaeval paintings show a much more realistic womanly mound. Similarly in the East a relaxed rounded belly is (or was) highly valued as a sign of spiritual achievement, the ability to operate in a grounded and centred way. Many people, both men and women, find it very hard to deliberately relax their bellies.

> **Exercise 14**
> Take a deep inbreath, letting it fill your tummy area, so that it visibly and tangibly expands with the breath (you may need to do a few pants with the diaphragm to loosen up first). Then breathe out, without pulling in your tummy. Try a few breaths like this, and see what sensations and feelings emerge. Focus on relaxing as many muscles in your lower torso as you can – including the sides and back.

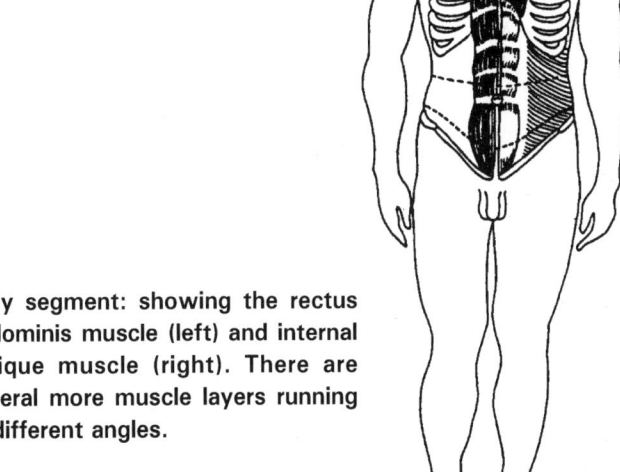

Belly segment: showing the rectus abdominis muscle (left) and internal oblique muscle (right). There are several more muscle layers running at different angles.

You will probably discover from this how closely your belly links with the diaphragm above and the pelvis below: muscles will stretch, and hopefully release, in both these areas as your belly expands. You can expect a few gurgles as well! Particularly important are the recti abdominus, two long rectus abdominis muscles (abs) that run down the belly from ribs to pelvis on either side of your navel – these seem to be linked by reflex with the sternocleidomastoids in the neck.

Gently massaging the belly area while breathing freely and easily can bring up all sorts of pains and emotions. Often there are specific sore spots carrying particular ideas and memories. The overall tone of the belly armour is frequently *tiredness:* old, tired grief; old, tired anger; old, tired fear. The emotions may have been curdling away down there for a very long time indeed.

But the belly, when it is alive and functioning, is an agent of release and elimination – it helps sort out the nourishing from the threatening, and channel each appropriately. As the belly 'wakes up' in bodywork, we hear all sorts of gurglings and rumblings – usually a sign of healthy activity as it resumes its functions of absorption and discharge. Gerda Boyesen worked for many years with the belly's wisdom. She found – as we have experienced for ourselves – that whenever the belly emits a particularly energetic gurgle, it signals some important thought, feeling or memory which may be below the threshold of awareness unless we take up the belly's cue and look within.

One particular set of feeling-memories in this segment is going to be about the cutting of the umbilical cord; there are usually very tender spots all around the navel that can restimulate this experience. It is also very closely linked with the waist segment – the shock of cutting the cord makes the diaphragm contract with a great gasp which is the first breath, so different from what that breath would have been had it been allowed to come naturally in its own time, with the umbilicus left to stop pulsing before it was severed.

For many people – perhaps more obviously for women in our culture – there is a particular issue around the relationship between mouth and belly. Appetite in one does not necessarily reflect hunger in the other: and often there is a good deal of confusion here, as we eat to satisfy all sorts of needs apart from bodily nourishment.

Among these needs can be the need to push feelings down out of awareness. Family mealtimes can be excruciating, and can set up a permanent association between eating, suppression and pain. A lot of us are so busy nibbling all day for the comfort of our mouths that we wouldn't recognise belly hunger if we encountered it. The poor, unloved, devalued belly has to bear the brunt of everything we shove down it. It needs restoring to its rightful and central role in the bodymind.

PELVIC SEGMENT

And so we arrive at the final section of the body armour – and an exceedingly important one. From the pelvis comes a whole other fundamental mode of relating to the world: our sexuality, which expresses itself in ways that cannot readily be turned into words. As Reich says, it is not really possible to attach a rational label to the expressive movements of the pelvis. Sexuality expresses *itself* rather than anything else, and its involuntary, mysterious quality is very frightening to the 'Spastic I'.

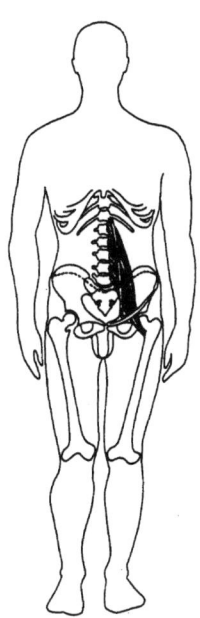

Pelvic segment: showing the psoas muscle

Before the pelvis can surrender to spontaneous sexual movement its armouring needs to be softened. This will release feelings that, although they often colour our lovemaking, are not essentially sexual in nature. Our pelvis often holds a good deal of fear and rage. This means that in lovemaking the easy soft swing takes on a frantic tone – either shoving and grinding, or moving very gingerly, like a person getting into a cold bath.

In Chapter 6 we shall be looking in more detail at this pelvic fear and rage, and considering how and why such emotions develop. For now, let's just notice that pelvic armouring has a deep effect on how we stand and walk; the legs and feet are so closely linked with the pelvis that we treat them as part of the same segment. If the pelvis is too stiff to sway freely as we move, there will be a corresponding stiffness and a brittle or numb feeling lower down. As Alexander Lowen says, sexual feeling to a great extent comes out of the ground, and our feet and legs need to be soft enough to let it rise.

> **Exercise 15**
>
> To help you understand what this means, stand with feet firmly planted and knees slightly bent and breathe down into the pit of your belly for a minute until everything has loosened up a little. Now explore the contact between the soles of your feet and the ground (this exercise is best done barefoot): shift your weight gently around your feet so the ground is massaging your soles. Now let your weight press down on the ball of one foot, as if taking a step forward – but don't take the step. What will happen is that your knee will start to straighten – but don't deliberately straighten the knee. Now your pelvis will want to rock forward and up: the impetus is transmitted from your energy exchange with the ground. Play with this movement for a while, using each leg in turn, and notice how important it is in graceful dancing – and think about how sexual dancing can be.

If our legs, feet and pelvis are relaxed, then there is a constant sense of exchange between ourselves and the ground: Mother Earth is really there under us, supporting and dialoguing with our bodymind. But not many of us feel this conversation much of the time. The process of learning to stand and walk, coinciding as it does with intense emotional events, has led us to cut off some sensation from our lower limbs – tensing knees, ankles, and hips in particular, and often twisting our legs out of alignment. We've learnt to 'stand up for ourselves', 'on our own two feet' – but at what price in missing flexibility and sensitivity?

Many of us have great unconscious terror of the ground, developed as we learnt to stand. This can show up in all the many phobias of snakes, mice, spiders, and so on – all fast-moving, ticklish, unstoppable creatures which we fear will run up our legs and into our bodies – like the earth energy itself and the uncontrollable feelings associated with it, including sexual ones. Other associated fantasies are those of the ground giving way, of quicksand, water and so on. There is often a fear of falling involved too – the ground seems a very long way down when we first pull ourselves erect.

In particular, our 'groundedness' or lack of it is connected with eye armouring. We may unconsciously try to hold on to the world with our eyes, rather than resting securely on our feet.

> **Exercise 16**
> Try closing your eyes, and really 'letting yourself down' into your feet: the sensation can be rather like entering water. Your knees will need to be loose and bent. Take a few steps, very slowly, with eyes still closed, and explore the sensation. Perhaps you feel as though you are going to fall over, or be hit. What do your arms want to do?

We have so far only looked at the front of the pelvis, the energy in and around our genital area. Also very important is the energy at the back, in our buttocks and anus, which may be extremely tight and tense. As we said in Chapter 2, children are very often pressured to control their bowels before they are naturally ready, before they are physically capable of closing the sphincters. So they learn to tense up the whole pelvic floor and buttocks in a desperate attempt to 'hold themselves in', 'pull themselves together'.

Such holding frequently becomes chronic and unconscious, leading to 'tight-arsed' attitudes in life, as we shall see in Chapter 6. A great deal of resentful hate is held here, which can take very brutal forms – both sadistic and masochistic – and involve a lot of stubbornness. This is a form of armouring that slows down our life energy and binds it in, and this sort of holding very much affects the energy in the back of our whole body.

The back of the body is our reservoir of strength: it's where we push from, where we hold on, support and endure. We can only be soft and open in the front if we feel strong and secure in the back. But this all depends on being able to 'dig our heels in' and transmit this solid strength through and up. A tight bum generally means that this flow gets stuck, and the backs of the legs will usually be tight too.

> **Exercise 17**
> Stand with feet a shoulder-width apart, and with your knees slightly bent. (Rigidly straight knees are a basic way of blocking off from the ground.) Join your hands loosely behind your back in an 'at ease' posture; now bend from the hips – not from the waist – and let gravity carry you as far forward as possible. Breathe easily, and let the outbreaths help you relax and lean further forward; visualise your sacrum moving gently upwards. The idea is that head, neck and back stay in the same straight line as when you were upright – you simply fold at the hinge of your hips.

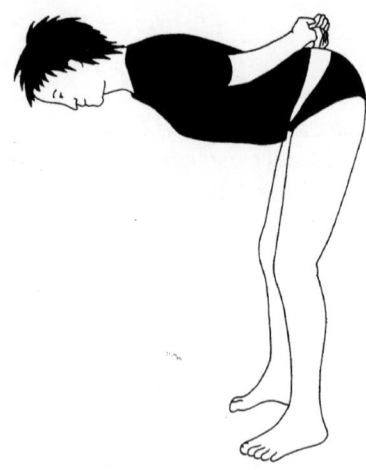

You will no doubt immediately feel a stretch on the backs of your legs, which can be quite painful. Don't strain yourself, just bend as far as you comfortably can, and if necessary hold the position for just a few seconds. It's important to breathe down into your belly as far as possible. With luck, if you maintain this position, your legs will start to tremble. This is splendid; it means that your muscle tension is letting go and your legs are lengthening, becoming literally more 'vibrant'. When you straighten up, still breathing into your belly and with knees loose, you may well feel a much deeper contact with the ground – almost as if your feet are sinking into the floor.

An important muscle joining up the whole pelvis, front and back, is the psoas, which runs on either side from the lower spine, right through the pelvis, and into the thighbone. This is the muscle that lets our pelvis rock back and forth in the orgasm reflex we described in the last chapter; often it is extremely tense and tight.

As we suggested, there is a strong relationship between looseness or tightness in the pelvis and in the jaw: this is one of the body's strongest reflexes, and an armoured jaw will stop the pelvis being free. It can be a bit of a bootstrap situation. Any release at either end creates a feedback of release at the other, and so on. We can even imagine a head superimposed on the pelvis, facing forwards but upside down: so that the chin coincides with the pelvic bone. Many other interesting relationships emerge – for instance, between nose and anus, so important for our learnt sense of disgust – often encouraging a tense pull-back of the face, away from 'down there'.

> **Exercise 18**
> The simplest possible exercise for checking out your pelvic segment is to stand with your knees loose, and rotate your hips as widely as you can – as if you were doing a hula dance. Keep breathing as you circle your pelvis first one way then the other; try large circles and very small ones, fast and slow movements, centring on one hip and then the other. But keep breathing!

Notice what you feel while doing the movement, and while standing still for a moment or so afterwards. Where else in your body are you aware of sensations?

Tension in the pelvis is likely to set up the conditions for ailments of the reproductive and eliminatory systems – piles, constipation or diarrhoea, thrush, cystitis, cervical cancer, period pains, and problems with the change of life.

GROUNDING, CENTERING, FACING

This, then, is the body in pieces: the body split up, in self-defence, into watertight compartments. Some segments are empty of charge, some overfull, some sour and stagnant, some at boiling point, some frozen, some yearning, some hidden and fearful. Before we move on to look at how character assembles itself out of these fragments, we want to suggest some unifying themes for the whole bodymind.

Three issues identified by David Boadella are Grounding, Centering and Facing, three capacities which help create our health and openness to the world. Grounding, we have already mentioned: this is our capacity to take a stand, to get a purchase on the world, to anchor ourselves ready to put out effort. Bodily grounding, a strong and flexible relationship with the earth and with gravity, corresponds to emotional grounding; one will not be found without the other. The grounded body says 'Here I am'; it takes a middle way between anxious stiff uprightness ('uptightness') and slumped inertia – a springy, reciprocal relationship with Mother Earth which draws on the depth and solidity of the ground for a sense of nourishment and belonging as well as for physical support. As Stanley Keleman puts it, 'if our relationship with the ground is tenuous, then our instinctual life and our body will also be tenuous. Our connection with the mystery of life will be tenuous.'

At times we need to ground ourselves in other ways: in relationships, in groups, in principles like loyalty and truth. The basis for all of these is a degree of freedom from armouring in feet, legs and pelvis; also in the buttocks, the back and shoulders, and in the head and neck. The more we look at grounding, the more we see how it involves a fundamental stance of the entire bodymind.

The same is true for centering, which is a capacity for wholeness and singleness in our bodymind. For most people the centre – or its absence – is around the solar plexus. If the diaphragm is too frozen with fear, then there will be a conscious or unconscious emptiness, a vacuum where the centre should be.

An armoured diaphragm splits the body into an upper and a lower half, cutting through unity. Like ungroundedness, it may relate to the severing of the umbilical cord – a sense of being cut off from the sources of nourishment and meaning.

For many people, there is also a sense of division between left and right sides, or between front and back, accompanied by deep, subtle twists in the posture. Thus grounding and centering are fundamentally linked; and we need both in order to face the world and other people, which we do with the whole front of our body, face, heart, belly and sex.

Facing is incomplete if our navel area feels empty and vulnerable, say, or if inadequate grounding puts a twist in our stance. If the eye segment is armoured then, as we have already indicated, there can be a sense of unreality and fragmentation. You may feel that you have no core or boundaries, that you are open to being invaded, swept off your feet, or leaking away. Thus these three capacities are very much intertwined with each other. We can only feel secure enough to open up and face the world if we are confident of our strength, the capacity to defend ourselves, which is embodied in our backs, shoulders and buttocks.

Then we can face things as they are, rather than as we would like them to be, and respond appropriately by opening or closing, reaching out or fending off, advancing or retreating. It is this capacity for appropriate action which armouring damages or eliminates entirely: it represents one form or another of compulsive defence. We are now going to look at the different blends and combinations of strategies for self-defence that make up the individual character.

5

Growing Up

> These children are not your children. They are the sons and daughters of life's longing for itself. You can strive to be like them. But you cannot make them just like you ...
>
> Kahlil Gibran, *The Prophet*
>
> We cannot solve life's problems except by solving them.
>
> M. Scott Peck, *The Road Less Travelled*

Facing things as they are is the essence of growing up: owning and using new capacities within ourselves; recognising and responding to new features of the world around us; coping realistically with the gains and losses to our well-being that these changes bring.

Or at least that's the idea. For many people, however, the phrase and the associated idea of 'growing up' carry such a mass of pain and anger that they will already have turned off from reading these words, and are responding by reflex. 'Why don't you grow up?' 'Stop being such a baby!' 'When I grow up I can do what I like, I'll understand everything and have power at last.' 'I don't ever want to grow up and be like *them*.'

Growing up, we suggest, is a process, not a state; we never reach a point of 'grown-upness', certainly not on our eighteenth birthday. Neither is being physiologically adult a measure of how much growing up we have managed to do. As children we are fed a lot of images of grown-upness that may seem both enticing – power, freedom, status, knowledge – and discouraging – conservatism, rigidity, responsibility, world-weariness. These are images and not reality, but of course they impose a certain reality on most of us. The process of growing up becomes one of growing into a set of shared beliefs and attitudes, many of which in our society are crippling.

Even in the healthiest environment there are always losses alongside the gains in skill and enjoyment which growing up brings. Apart from anything else there is the simple loss of *familiarity*, which we tend to equate with security. However limiting and impoverished a particular situation may be, we are at least surviving it, and it's often tempting to choose the frying pan rather than the fire, a known and survivable limitation rather than an unknown mixture of promise and threat.

So it's a genuine question: do we *want* to grow up? Physically, we may have little choice – the first great example is the foetus who simply grows too big for the womb to hold it, and our growth process continues with the same irresistibility (though some people do seem to keep a 'childlike', underdeveloped physique which perhaps corresponds to an emotional unwillingness to grow up). As far as feeling and behaviour go, however, we can choose at any point to stop, not to pass through the next gateway in our developmental process. Although we apparently continue with life, our being has said 'No' on a deep level: inwardly we are committed to preserving the attitudes and values of the past.

In childhood, this refusal is clearly not literal. We can't, for example, go on breastfeeding for our whole life. But we *can* go on manifesting the attitudes which are appropriate to the breastfeeding or bottle-feeding period and which, if maintained, become negative and unhelpful. Genuine dependence turns into clinging, weedy behaviour; we act as if the world owes us a living. (And, of course, we can take up a different sort of bottle, or other comforting drugs, as adults.)

This is quite different from the way in which one stage can and should act as a *foundation* for the next. To continue the breastfeeding example, we should be able to build on the secure feeling that we can be fed by the universe, as breastfeeding itself builds on the deep security of the previous experience of being continuously nurtured through the umbilical cord. We move from continuous, effortless feeding into a situation of dependence on a reliable source of nourishment, where we become more and more capable of actively asking for it. Thus by stages we move gradually into the adult situation of having to seek out and create our own nourishment. If all goes well there is a safe and gradual progression, even if there are some difficult moments, like weaning, or adolescence.

Growing up isn't just about childhood. True, it is most obvious and intense early in life, but the *opportunities* to grow continue throughout our existence. Physically, our body goes on changing and developing both emotionally and mentally. We face new situations which challenge us to respond in new ways, to reconsider ourselves and reintegrate our values. How we cope with these opportunities depends a great deal on what has happened in our childhood, because by the time we are physical adults most of us have made some basic decisions *not* to go on changing. At one or more of the crucial developmental thresholds, we have rejected the new in favour of the old; not through wilfulness or inadequacy, but because our world did not give us the necessary support in a deeply scary and demanding situation. (It may also be that elements of our genetic inheritance predispose us to avoid certain developmental paths and prefer others.)

As we have already suggested, these 'decisions not to change' are what creates armouring. Once made, such choices are not easy to unmake, especially since we are normally unaware of having made them. They are frozen into the basic pattern of our bodymind; secretly, tenaciously, they warp our responses to every new situation, enforcing a particular style of limitation of our bodily and emotional mobility.

We may be unable to raise our arms easily over our head, for example – unable to ask for help. Or we may be unable to push our jaw forward – and to defy authority; unable to balance on one leg – and to feel securely grounded in the world.

There are limitless examples, but as we shall see they tend to be organised within each person into a few basic patterns, a few main styles of defending against the world and our own impulses, each relating to a major threshold of development over which we stumbled in childhood. We use 'character' as the name for these patterns – for the inflexible, protective structures built into our ways of being in the world; the armoured bodymind which people often falsely identify with the real self.

The irony is that many of the attitudes which physical adults hold up to the young as examples of 'grown-upness' are in fact pieces of character armouring. The caution, the conventionality, the exaggerated politeness and deep habitual patterns which are supposed to indicate 'maturity' are really more like the first stages of death. Young people who instinctively recognise this shrink in horror from the cold rigidity of adults, retreating into destructive nihilism – 'I'm never going to grow up'.

Armouring forms different patterns in each person; each of us favours some styles of expression and of holding more than others. In a very real and remarkable way our armouring presents a fossilised history of its own development: old feelings that have turned to stone, layer upon frozen layer, like the rings of some prehistoric tree. It is possible systematically to bring these fossil feelings back to life, liberating the energy that is trapped in holding them down – trapped in the past.

It's a great help in this task of creative archaeology to realise that character, though differently constructed for each person, falls into patterns. We can look at a particular way of relating to the world, of holding tension in the body, and connect it with other similar patterns, and so approach the individual with some sense of what feelings are being frozen and why, some idea of which era of childhood the process relates to. Of course, we can never deny that person's uniqueness, the very uniqueness we are trying to help them liberate, but the *armour*, as distinct from the human being within it, will almost always fit into one of relatively few patterns.

There are many different ways in which theorists can and do classify character for purposes of recognition – and no way to say that one is 'right' and another 'wrong'. It's like sorting buttons: we can put all the red ones together, or all the ones with four holes, or all the wooden ones – it depends entirely on what we are aiming to do with the buttons. We can, however, point out the different values which different modes of character analysis hold up as 'normal' and 'healthy'. What do they think human beings are 'really' like?

Some approaches to grouping character are attempting to say something about the origin and function of the attitudes involved: what they protect against, for example, and why. We feel that these approaches are powerful and potentially useful, for they have direct implications about how character can be melted and loosened. But at the same time they are dangerous, because if we go off at the wrong angle we are likely to miss the real person completely, and because they create the possibility of manipulating individual personality into what we regard as 'good for them'. Our own work with character starts from the belief and experience that human beings are originally and fundamentally loving; that our primal impulses are for contact and creativity; and that character armour represents our response to the *frustration* of these original impulses. So rather than trying to 'turn people into' healthy and loving beings, we are trying to help them melt the layers which obscure their original healthy and loving nature.

Of course, it's a rare individual whose character consists of one pure type, who reacts all the time to every situation along the same groove. Generally, each character can be seen as a complex interweaving of strands, often with many layers of defences lying 'on top of' each other, so that as one dissolves the next comes into view.

These layers represent phases of historical development in each person, ways of reacting which get frozen into us in a sequence of attitudes. Thus, in a crude example, there might be a layer of frozen fear which the person protects with violent anger, and then covers *this* up with a sneering politeness, which she tries to control with a stance of sweet reason – and so on.

Reich saw each of us as consisting of three major layers which show up in our character attitudes and in our musculature. He referred to these as Core, Middle Layer, and Surface. The Core is our 'original mind', as Buddhists sometimes call it: our innate, organic capacity for love and creative work. For an infant growing up in our society, her attempts to express her core nature, to move this loving and enthusiastic energy outwards, are often met with systematic coldness and repression. Love, by its nature, turns to anger when frustrated, the organism's way of focusing energy on blasting through whatever obstructs its satisfaction.

But if this anger is *itself* suppressed, we end up with a superficial layer of socialised 'niceness' covering up all sorts of hateful and vicious feelings, created out of anger which cannot discharge itself, stewing and stagnating under the Surface. It is this Middle Layer which many people take to be their 'real innermost self' – a terrifying idea, which naturally enough makes them feel they must stay concealed at all costs!

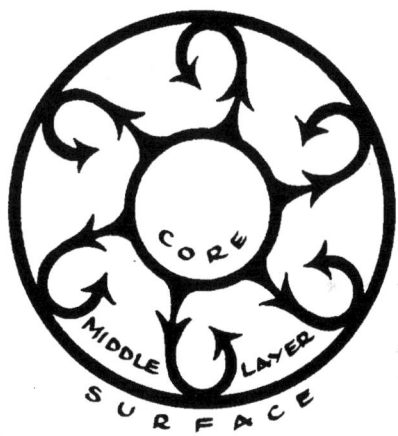

A dim awareness of the Middle Layer, without any direct sense of the Core, is what stops a lot of people from working at their own growth. 'If I let go of my control I might attack people with an axe, or have sex in the middle of the road' is a common attitude. The Core may be seen as if it is outside ourselves rather than inside, so that goodness is in *other* people, or in Heaven. Will I like what I find? Will other people like it? Am I *normal*? These are the fears that police our separation from our own core nature.

Character defends against outside threats ('they won't like it'); but equally, or even more importantly, it defends against inside feelings which seem too dangerous to express or even to acknowledge ('I won't like it').

Hate and violence, though, are only a distorted version of love and pleasure. Once we contact our original nature, with its primary feelings of wholesomeness, we can find the courage to release what Reich called 'secondary emotions' without feeling overwhelmed by them. Of course, to contact the Core we need to explore some of the Middle Layer which is in the way, so it is a delicate process of opening up as much as we dare, and seeing that we gain a tremendous amount from doing so. At the same time our Core offers a natural self-regulation of how much we open up at any given moment. Once again, our feelings are not the problem, but our feelings *about* our feelings most certainly are.

This is particularly true when the feeling is of guilt, manifesting itself in a belief that our defensive character structure is 'our fault'. But we are not to blame for our decisions to 'never grow up'; and nor, really, is anyone else. Everybody at all times does their best; all energy starts out from the clear core and struggles to reach expression. If we have decided to say 'no' to some of life's demands, it was always the result of an accurate judgement that we couldn't handle them – *at that time*.

However, circumstances have changed. As adults our potential powers and capacities have greatly increased, and it would probably make sense to revise some of those past decisions. One thing this means is becoming *conscious* of them – re-owning the frozen history of our character armour.

So what stopped us growing up?

No single incident will bind us into a straitjacket of character armouring. Often a single incident becomes the focus, and this may emerge in the course of therapy, sometimes with stunning force. But that memory usually stands as a symbol for the whole *context* in which we grew up – or rather, failed to do so. We recall one occasion on which our anger, say, was swallowed back through fear of adult power. But if it only happened once we could easily cope with it – it's the constant repetition of swallowed anger that creates the adult character unable not only to express anger but even consciously to feel it.

As we have said, the whole purpose of armouring is to remove conflict from consciousness. We could see this as a sort of *learning*, not very different in principle from the way we learn to walk or to talk, so that the actual mechanics of the operation become automatic and unconscious: we 'just do it'. In the case of armouring, though, it's the tensing of the muscles to *prevent* action (including breathing) that becomes automatic, coupled with the equivalent mental 'act' of blanking out thoughts and feelings.

Tension in a particular muscle system will tend to produce *more* tension as the muscles shorten to fit in with how they are being used. A wider range of muscles thus becomes affected, so that eventually the movement we are inhibiting tends to become physically impossible, a defensive habit imprinted on the body, just as it becomes mentally 'impossible' to feel and express the repressed emotions. Changes take place in the sheaths of connective tissue that surround our muscles. What started off as *doing* – tensing muscles as a deliberate act – has become a state of *being:* 'that's just the way I am'.

We are going to show how these character patterns – 'just the ways we are' – emerge out of specific stages of development that we all go through, and which in turn correspond to specific areas and organs of the body. These patterns, found in particular segments of our armour, first formed during the phase of childhood when our energy was focused in that area of the body, a result of the work of growing up that was going on there. The body armour is a map of character – but an *archaeological* map.

In the womb, the embryo grows from the head down. This is the direction of the energy stream around which we develop. After birth, the process is repeated on another level in our formative interactions with the world. The energy of our need, our interest, our desire, streams through one body system after another, tracing in the first few years of life a path down the body from head to pelvis. This is partly a metaphor, but to a remarkable extent – as we shall see – it is a simple statement of fact.

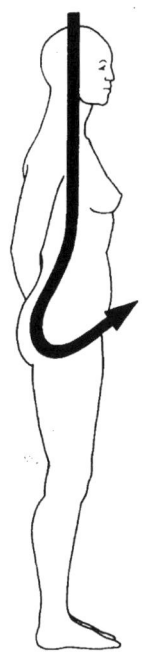

Clearly there are many 'stages of growth' – as many as we choose to name – but our system of character analysis focuses on some main stages relating to those parts of the body where we 'exchange energy' with the universe: places where we take things in and give things out – and which are, therefore, sites of pleasure and frustration, satisfaction and loss. These parts surround what we call the 'heartlands' of the body: our torso and belly, the inner areas of which, the great involuntary muscles of the heart, the diaphragm and the intestines, we can identify on a bodily level with the Core. The word 'core' in fact comes from the Latin for 'heart' and there is a very special relationship between the heart segment and our primary feelings of love, contact and creativity.

Thus the places where character is defined are the places where energy moves between the heartlands of our body and the outside world: eyes, mouth, chest, anus and genitals are the main systems involved, with other areas like legs, throat and back taking their cue from the sorts of charge, blocking and investment that happen at the head, tail and heart of the organism. Armouring elsewhere will give a particular 'flavour' to the character, but it is what happens in the head, tail and heart that defines the essential character attitude.

Since we all go through much the same biological process of growing up, we have all experienced the essential attitude towards the world that goes along with each character type. These attitudes are all part of a healthy life function; we all need an energetic connection with seeing and thinking, with feeding and speaking, with self-regulation, assertion and love. And each of us emerges from childhood with an entirely healthy preferred style of being, based in one or more of these core attitudes.

What keeps us stuck in *negative* versions of these attitudes is when some of our growth energy is still trapped back in that phase of our development, never having satisfactorily resolved the issues that arose there. At each stage we need help, validation and support from the world. Without these, a certain part of us never makes it through to the next stage: like Peter Pan, we just can't face growing up.

That part of us will then tend to identify every new situation which comes along as being nothing but a new version of that same issue from the past. So, to use the same example as earlier, someone who hasn't properly dealt with the experience of being weaned will see every new person in their life as a potential provider or withholder of nourishment – 'Are you my Mummy?' is the constant unconscious question. Every crisis of life will then be understood as being basically a threat to nourishment, whatever the actual issues may be. The process of creative learning, whereby we use the past to draw lessons for the future, has here gone out of control. In a sense no future exists, only action replays of the past. We will return to some of these issues in Chapter 10.

The same sorts of pattern correspond to each phase of development over the first few years of life, up to the point at which our basic character is pretty well formed. To each bodily function of exchange with the world there corresponds a basic *need*, which must be satisfied before the bodymind can fully move on. Insofar as that need is denied or left unsatisfied, a part of our life force is 'left behind' in the form of muscular armour and character structure, and future issues will be comprehended largely in terms of that unmet need. For the eyes it is the sense of existence and reality; for the mouth, feeding and support; for the chest, validation; for the anus, grounding and self-management; and for the genitals, assertiveness, play and surrender.

The great majority of us have to some basic extent made it through to the end of the process, the beginning of independent life, with the ability to be open, accept reality, and have genital sexual relationships. Bruised and battered, tattered and torn, we've made it – but not completely. We've left a considerable part of our potential power and pleasure back in those growth stages, locked up in the armouring that forms around our frustrations.

We can only fully let go to reality and pleasure, it seems, when we replay and release this old history, to own our existence, nourishment, validation, self-regulation, assertiveness and play. What we then achieve is the *wholeness* of our bodymind from top to toes, able to focus and express itself through each and every organ, able to carry on with the open-ended process of growing.

We can achieve a relationship of wholeness with our entire developmental process. There is a perfectly healthy 'regression' that goes on all the time: every night we return to a womb-like state to sleep and dream, and at different moments in our daily life we are using the attitudes and feelings appropriate to every phase of life. Even a six-month-old baby can at times be seen regressing to earlier phases for reassurance and comfort. And there is also a process of what, in contrast to regression, we might call 'progression' along our lifeline – the times when we feel old as the hills, or when a child suddenly shows unexpectedly adult attitudes. This is all a natural part of being alive. The important thing is to have the capacity for free movement, rather than being compelled to enter or stay in a particular state.

It is our character structure which can make some forms of 'release therapy' very disappointing after a while. It's a tremendous relief to cry, to rage, to scream and to shake, especially if we have spent years being unable to do so. But eventually it is brought home to us that there has been only a limited change in our ways of living our life; that we still have most of the problems we came with, and we don't seem to have *that* much less need to discharge emotion. (Often people think this need should go away; but it is a basic human function like eating or excreting, and doesn't go away.)

Our character is like a sponge which soaks up and holds on to certain kinds of feeling. It's comparatively easy – and very important – to learn how to let those feelings go, like squeezing out the sponge. In itself, however, this won't alter *the structure of the sponge:* it will soak up the same feelings again at the first opportunity. Working to change the character itself is a much harder and more subtle task. In the following chapters we shall show how we go about it.

6

Character Positions

> Most people have very little tendency to look at their character objectively.
>
> Wilhelm Reich, *Character Analysis*

We shall now work down the body again, as we did in the chapter on the segments, but this time looking only at the head, tail and heart 'energy exchange' segments. Freudians call the head and tail areas 'erogenous zones'. We add to these the heart segment, which also reaches out to exchange energy with the world. We shall describe the sort of character attitudes which accompany a serious block in each segment. In this way we will set up some caricature figures, stiffer and more one-dimensional than almost any real person, but from a blend of which, and influenced by armouring elsewhere in the body, our individual character is formed.

We call these attitudes character *positions* to emphasise the fact that, for most people, they manifest only at certain times and in certain conditions. Most of us are pretty healthy and creative in our best moments, though even at these times we may tend to show a certain *style* of creativity that reflects a favoured character position. We may be better at standing our ground than at flowing, for example, because of an emphasis on the 'holding' position, or we may be better at looking after than at being looked after because of unresolved oral feelings. At other, more stressful, moments we may get stuck in the less creative versions of these same character positions: compelled to try and hold our feelings in, perhaps, or feeling totally weak and unable to function independently.

All of this should become clearer as we go along. The main point is that each of us contains within us the potential for *each* character position, because they take their being from life experiences we have all had. The specific events of our individual lives, however, determine which one or two or three positions are strongest in us, because we have had the most difficulty crossing those particular developmental thresholds.

In each segment we can see two different kinds of block, one based on *yearning* and the other on *denial* of that yearning. To use an example from the last chapter, someone may be eternally looking for nourishment ('are you my Mummy?'), or, in a further act of repression they may be eternally pretending that there is no such need, and closing down their energy flow so as to numb their feelings. These repressed feelings will come out indirectly in one way or another, however, perhaps in the end as a physical symptom. In order to dissolve this 'denying block', it must turn back into a 'yearning' one; that is, the individual must become aware of the need they are repressing as the first stage towards letting go of it. In this example, the hard clenched jaw must become a soft sucking one.

Character positions fall easily into two groups: those organised around armouring in the head, and those organised around armouring in the pelvis. Head segment characters tend to be *under-grounded* in their attitudes – 'up in the air' in one way or another – while pelvic segment characters tend to be *over-grounded*, rigid and immobile or flooded with earth energy. The heart segment stands between these two extremes, and is concerned with *facing*.

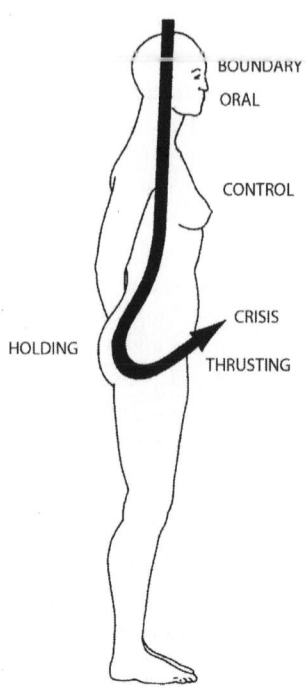

The terms used for the character positions are mainly our own, rather than those used by Reich or by other schools of psychotherapy describing essentially similar ways of seeing character. We have developed new names because we see the orthodox ones either as abusive ('Masochistic', 'Passive Feminine'), confusing, or over-technical.

As already mentioned, we are following a sequence which moves down the body from the scalp and eyes, following a sequence of development through the early years of childhood. We can visualise an energy path which crosses through the body at the waist from front to back as it moves from the heart and chest to the anus; and then curves back up through the pelvis to the front of the body and the genitals.

BOUNDARY POSITION

Eye segment block: issues of *existence*

In the first days of our life outside the womb, we urgently seek contact with those who care for us. We need to receive unspoken messages which tell us 'Yes, you're here, you exist, I recognise and care for you'; to see and be seen, touch and be touched, hear and be heard. The focus for this affirmation that we exist seems to be the whole skin surface of our bodies, and more specifically, the upper head and particularly the eyes.

We are not really describing anything mysterious here; you can see parents and babies instinctively drinking deep in each others' eyes right from the start, especially during feeding, and there have been several studies of how badly affected a baby is if the parent keeps turning their attention away. The same happens if she is not held and stroked enough – enough to feel *real*.

We depend utterly on this fundamental validation, and if we don't get it at the start of life through our eyes and skin, there will be a long-term incompleteness and fragility built into our bodymind development. A part of our energy will stay back in those first days of life, still seeking that primary contact which says 'you exist'. This insecurity can be seen in the eyes of the adult, and sensed in their interaction with the world. At least part of the character will be built upon a basic uncertainty about their own wholeness and reality, and every crisis of life will be experienced as a threat to *being*.

If the person stays in the same family situation this lack of warm human contact in earliest infancy is likely to be continued in childhood, and may be reinforced by frightening or confusing experiences that need to be shut out of awareness. This kind of history puts a particular stress on *boundaries*. Do I have any? Where are they? Is it safe to let anything come through them? These are very real questions for someone with a strong eye segment block. With a 'yearning block', someone will feel a lack of wholeness. They may experience themselves as 'in bits', fragmented, 'all over the place', liable under pressure to flee or fall apart. There will be a drive to find some form of the missing primary contact: 'I must see, I must understand', a compulsion to make sense of things, to find an answer. There will be a 'seeking', intense expression in the eyes, which can be frightening to other people whose own deep feelings are sparked off by this demand for contact.

Does this sound familiar? It is partly this need to understand which draws someone to read – or to write – about the structures of the bodymind. You may also recognise in yourself the 'denying eye block', which seeks to repress this frightening need for contact, understanding and validation. Its message is 'I can't or won't see or understand'. The fear of what's out there, or what's inside, is so great that the person closes down their perception in some way, clouds or fogs or confuses, 'goes away in the eyes' as Reich puts it.

A small example is the otherwise sensible person who 'just can't see' some area of reality. Because of our training, for women it is often mathematics or mechanics; for men, it can be emotions. We can't understand it because it stirs up too much: we cannot bear to keep our attention on it and re-experience the anger, say, of being put down in childhood, or the anguish in our own heart. For many people, psychic and spiritual realities fall into this category: 'I won't look because there's nothing there.'

On a wider scale, the denying eye block puts people severely out of touch with the world and with other humans. They feel 'cut off', 'unreal', but may well be giving out conscious or unconscious messages of 'stay away'; a coldness and an invisible wall which is their response to intolerable *fear*.

Fear is very much the key emotion for the boundary character position: fear of being overwhelmed, of exploding or imploding, of one's fragile foothold on existence crumbling. A source of denying eye blocking is very often the need, as a child, to escape adult scrutiny, to not be seen *into*. There is a lack of fundamental confidence which means a natural boundary between inside and outside fails to develop, so that a harsh and exaggerated cut-off is created in its place.

A good sign that we are occupying the boundary position is if we become confused about what is *outside* and what is *inside*. Perhaps we find ourselves seeing other people as feeling angry or afraid when that is what *we* are feeling, or perhaps we let other people's ideas take us over and dominate our own sense of things. Or maybe we mix up one kind of reality with another, mistaking our own energy for some sort of psychic or science-fiction 'attack' from outside.

All these experiences are seen in orthodox psychiatry as reflecting 'schizoid' character structures. This is *not* the same thing as 'schizophrenia' but, one might say, a very mild version of the problems for which that label is used. These are the sorts of experiences described so well in R.D. Laing's earlier books, like *The Divided Self*. In a sense, though, Laing perpetuates the split he describes by writing only about the *mind*, and not the body. This is one boundary that tends to exist very strongly in such characters.

Eye segment blocking makes it hard to live in the body – one form it can take, as we have already noted, is the 'ivory tower' intellectual. It also makes it hard to achieve wholeness; the bodies of people with strong boundary characters often have an unfinished or unintegrated look to them – different parts may give contradictory messages. Sometimes there is a childlike, undeveloped physique, perhaps the large head and spindly neck of the baby who in essence is still present, still seeking wholeness and validation. Someone really stuck in the boundary position will give off a deep sense of 'wrongness' with their bodymind; other people may instinctively tend to avoid them, which of course reinforces their isolation and fear.

Another form which this 'flight from the body' often takes is an extreme sensitivity to, and interest in, the 'psychic', 'spiritual' realm. However, because the boundary position is severely under-grounded, their very real sensitivity is quite undiscriminating. Genuine contact gets mixed up with complete fantasy, often projecting the person's own feelings and sensations 'out there' on to other people or 'spirits'. The awareness of energy, however confused, is real and strong; in particular, the boundary character will often be strongly conscious of the energy field surrounding the body – the 'aura'.

It is important to see how the needs and concerns of the boundary position – as with every other character – are basically quite rational and universal. Every baby passes through a phase of contacting the world and other people through eyes, ears, nose and skin, and a phase of setting boundaries, making a sense of self which is secure against outside invasion or 'leaking'. Every adult can develop out of this 'eye energy' a creative enjoyment of looking, thinking, discovery, eye contact, flirting, visions, inspiration and meditation.

What we are calling an eye block, a boundary position, is a state where someone has not yet fully managed to create a basis for this adult creativity. They are still partially stuck in an early childhood crisis, and are reducing adult experience to these terms. By their very sensitivity, though, they are many of our artists, our mediums, our prophets, our seers.

Exercises to give a direct experience of the character positions necessarily involve working with another person, since the positions are fundamentally about relationship. If you have a friend with whom you feel happy to try it, then the following exercise should put you in touch with your boundary material (for the idea of these exercises and some specific details, we are grateful to Helen Davis):

> **Exercise 19**
> Person A, stand with your back close up against a wall, pressing yourself against it and coming up on tiptoe, so your whole posture is 'up and away'. Opening your eyes very wide, breathe high in your chest, without ever fully emptying your lungs. Person B, stand a few feet away, and holding eye contact, slowly advance on A. Person A, experiment with saying things like 'No', 'keep away', and so on; let yourself go into the feelings that come up.
>
> After a few minutes, stop, make contact and remind yourselves who each other really is, share what happened, and try the exercise in reverse.

ORAL POSITION

Jaw segment block: issues of *feeding and support*

The primary infant experience connected with our mouths is breast- or bottle-feeding. At its best this is an experience of profound contentment and pleasure, the nearest thing to getting back inside the womb, reuniting with the mother's body. That floating, drifting, relaxed dreaminess is often maintained long into childhood with thumb sucking, comfort blankets and so on. It is also a crucial component of our adult well-being. If all goes well we grow up with the secure conviction that the universe can nourish and support us, that there will be good times, that life is fundamentally *possible*. This conviction enables us to move out effectively into the world. We can mobilise our energies because at other times we are able to let go and be supported.

For very many people, though, the weaning process and infant feeding will have been disturbed and damaged in some way. This is not really anyone's *fault* – there is so much guilt in this area! It is very hard – though not totally impossible – for us as parents to give our children more than we had ourselves; the mother or father with distress around feeding and support issues will have difficulties in making their own child feel secure.

Of course, the parents may have real problems in their own current life, or simply too much to do, distracting them from giving full attention to the baby. Their own instincts may have been distorted by bizarre 'expert' theories of when and how to feed. The birth of more children may speed up the weaning process, together with the closely related process of 'standing on your own feet', which is often beyond what the child can handle.

The 'oral yearning' character position, then, seeks to be *fed*. The whole message emanating from the person is 'feed me, hold me up'. There is often a sense of physical weakness; a thin, stringy, weedy body like a plant deprived of light, which has bolted and stretched itself out – the child eternally reaching to be picked up and cuddled. Less commonly, there is the fat oral character, with a jolly grin concealing their resentful, sadistic determination to chew up and devour the whole world.

With the oral position there is almost always an aggressive edge, a profound bitterness. Why won't people look after me? How can they expect me to fend for myself in this cold, cruel world? Can't they see how important and special I am? In the oral position, we tend to be 'on strike', withdrawing our labour from life in the hope that people will see how unfairly we are being treated. Sulking, in other words!

The infantile nature of these attitudes is very obvious, and often very irritating. Part of the irritation, though, is that we are uncomfortably reminded of feelings we have ourselves. Rare is the person who, as a child, felt fully satisfied and nurtured; who spontaneously initiated their own weaning and every other stage of their independence; who truly feels they have had *enough*. When we refer to feelings as 'infantile', we must remember that they are fully appropriate for infants to have: we *did* need looking after, we *were* special and important.

Many of us, in order to survive, have developed a 'denying oral' block, contradicting our needs. We present clenched teeth, stiff lips – the Clint Eastwood, 'strong silent type'. Here is a fundamental stance of 'I won't' – eat, cry, ask, speak, get angry – reveal myself as needy and yearning.

Alongside oral blocks we often notice an *irritability* that is both emotional and physical – a peculiar hot prickliness to the skin, and a general difficulty in becoming comfortable. It is as if the person's teeth are being set on edge, and teething can be a very serious factor in developing an oral position. Suppressed anger commonly comes out in 'biting', 'sharp-tongued' speech. There is a big overlap between weaning, teething, standing and learning to talk, often with a lot of tension around trying to ask for or demand the feeding we need, trying to articulate the unfairness we are experiencing.

The child may grow up to be a smooth, glib talker, with many rationalisations for their dependence on others – a 'sponger' or a con artist. Or – and sometimes at the same time – she may be caught in a trap, since expressing the rage she feels just makes adults withdraw even more, so that she feels forced to 'bite it back', 'swallow it down'. Stammering is one possible result of this contradiction – 'I can't (mustn't) say what I want to say' – so is tight-lipped silence. The discomfort already referred to may mean 'It isn't *right!*'

You may have already noticed how people often react against their real character so as to conceal it; what we can call a 'flip' into a polar opposite position. With the oral position, there is often a tendency to become a 'compulsive carer', someone who looks after everyone in sight – whether they like it or not. We can recognise this attitude by the absence of open-hearted love. People in this position are often the social workers and official carers from whom everyone runs a mile! What such people need to recognise is that in caring for others they are secretly acting out what they want for themselves, yet their caring is undermined by the concealed aggression and resentment of the oral position.

Oral blocking, as we have said, makes it difficult to feel fundamentally secure in the world. While the boundary character often feels unreal, in danger of annihilation, the oral character is real and here in the world, but often terribly lonely, empty and cold. 'Empty' is the key word: an inner gulf, an absence of energy for self-starting or carrying through projects. No petrol in the tank; no milk in the tummy! Most of us have at least occasional experiences of this state.

An oral block will interfere with full enjoyment of activities like eating, drinking, talking, kissing, singing. We will either dislike them, or compulsively over-indulge them – always the two fundamental tactics for dealing with any kind of stuckness. The yearning oral character can try to fill herself up with almost anything: food, drink, TV, music, drugs, sex, ideas, or looking after other people!

When oral energy is freed, it expresses itself creatively in an *appetite for life*, a capacity for gusto and enjoyment including, but not restricted to, the sorts of oral activities described above. Often there is a genuine eloquence, which can serve other functions than wheedling. In particular there is a genuine concern with *justice*, that no one be left out or rejected, and a true capacity to nurture others, based on a sense of security in oneself.

Exercise 20

To experience your oral position, work with person B standing on a chair, and person A reaching up to them with their arms and their whole body – again, tending towards tiptoe. Breathe fairly deeply, one breath at a time, with pauses at the end of the inhale and the exhale. Person A says things like 'Please', 'Play with me', 'Feed me', while person B experiments with 'No', 'Not now', 'Leave me alone'. After a while stop, make contact, and reverse roles.

CONTROL POSITION

Heart segment block: issues of *validation*

A good experience of the oral position means that we have felt enough support from those caring for us to move forward into a more independent role in the world. Small children want to start playing 'away from' their parent – but still in visual range, with the sense of being seen and validated: 'Did you see me on the swings, dad?' Support is still crucial, but less *direct* than in the oral stage: the child is being held, not by the arms of the carer, but by their attention and their acknowledgement of the child's experience.

Through the kinds of experiences we – hopefully – have at this stage, we are learning about 'other minds': learning that other people exist, that they have roughly the same kinds of experiences we do, and that we can project ourselves imaginatively into their experience as they can into ours. Through play – especially play in which we are held in the parent's gaze, and play in which we ourselves 'control' and 'manipulate' the parent ('Now you be the baby, and you're sad because the mummy's not there, and then I'm the mummy and I come back ...') – we develop a sense of 'mental space', of an inner world, and that other people also have inner worlds. Through adults' support of our play and fantasy, we learn to engage with an interpersonal reality.

What can go wrong at this point is that, instead of our experience being supported, it can be *denied*. The important adults don't join in with us, don't let us be at the centre of a playful interpersonal space. This may be simply because they are themselves tired, drained and emotionally preoccupied. Or they may have a compulsion to dominate, 'You will do what I say and like it'. Or often they are caught up in a mistaken kind of caring, which is deeply undermining of our reality: 'You don't really mean that, dear'; 'Of course you're not sad, nothing to be upset about'; 'There's mummy's brave boy'. All these sorts of interactions masquerade as contact, but are actually profoundly out of contact with the child's true experience.

These reactions to our need for supported play hurt our heart. It becomes bruised, frozen, withered, numbed. On another level, it also damages our cognitive development, and prevents us from learning about the existence of other selves – from learning to empathise. Ultimately, we may give up on any expectation that contact with other people will be *possible*, that anyone will see and hear and touch our reality. Yet we still have needs, of course; how are we to get them met?

Really only two techniques lie open to someone whose heart and mind have been blocked in this way. We can seek to *dominate* other people, by physical force or by force of will; or we can seek to seduce and *manipulate* them. (These options each relate to another later character position, as we will see.) Underlying either strategy is a fundamental lack of belief that other people are *real*, that they have feelings and needs, experience pain and pleasure. It is as if we have been stranded on a planet of androids, and have to learn the codes by which they can be controlled and made to serve us. This is the aspect of the control position which has led some therapists to label it 'psychopathic': if other people are androids, we can feel free to cheat them, hurt them, even kill them.

This belief stems, of course, from feeling treated like an android ourselves; it stems from other people's apparent lack of belief in our reality. We are seeking *revenge*. (We are also stuck in repeating what was originally an age-appropriate need to be in charge and the centre of attention.) And yet there is no satisfaction in that revenge: our victories over others are without savour, because they fail to meet our underlying yearning for empathy, for heart-to-heart contact, for the recognition of our needs. If we deny that yearning, we are left with the option of hiding ourselves behind a 'false self', an outer persona which acts at being caring and loving and good, while inside we are silently saying to ourselves 'keep quiet, don't show anything, keep your head down, stay safe ...'.

The jammed-up heart of the control character usually manifests physically as a sense of bulkiness and inflatedness in their upper torso, especially in the yearning version: their chest is pushed out in a dumb show of domination, like a cartoon sergeant-major or society dowager. They are often fleshy in a rather smooth way, and there can be a shark-like mirthless grin permanently in place. Mussolini's bodily appearance is an exaggeration of the control position.

But of course very few people in this position are Mussolinis, or psychopaths. More generally, they are struggling with difficulties around making contact and directly expressing need: sometimes closer to recognising other people as real, sometimes further away. Creative use of control energy comes out in *leadership*, in being able to take responsibility for group needs. Control characters can be wonderful hosts, the life and soul of the party, able to remember everyone's name and favourite food; they can be charismatic performers, basking in the love of the audience and able to repay that love by making everyone feel good. The potential downside of this is the contempt that leaders or entertainers can feel for the crowd; the cold calculation behind the host or hostess's smile.

The heart centre plays a very special role in the human energy system: in many ways we could see all of the character positions as representing different ways in which the heart tries to express itself. So the control character with their locked-up heart is wounded in a very deep place. But always, the wound represents the potential for growth: people whose energy focuses in the control position are people whose energy focuses in their heart – people with 'big hearts', with the capacity for big expression, the capacity to look after others, to have 'the whole world in their hands'. What is often harder for them is to be looked after themselves: to balance out their bigness by daring to feel *small*.

> **Exercise 21**
> Person A stand with knees bent, leaning forward from the waist with back arched so that head is upright; arms stretched forward in front of you. (This is very uncomfortable. If it feels easy, you're not doing it right.) Person B stands in front, just out of reach. Person A tells B what is happening for them – e.g., 'my back's hurting' – and person B systematically denies everything they say – e.g., 'No it isn't, you're fine', not forgetting 'I'm not contradicting you/ignoring what you say'. Continue for as long as you can bear it, then make contact and reverse.

HOLDING POSITION

Anal block: issues of *self-regulation*

Now we move to the other end of the torso, and the other arena of our energy exchange with the world: the pelvis. Here the next big issue that creates character arises around learning to control our own bodily functions, in particular those related to what we take into and out of our bodies. For most of us the key event is toilet training; learning to recognise the sensations of full bowel or bladder, and to respond in the appropriate way at the appropriate time and place.

Acquiring these skills is a great milestone in our development, and can go along with a tremendous new sense of power and worth as we are gently encouraged and praised by the adults around us. It's part of identifying with our own bodymind, and its natural processes and rhythms. More often, though, the impatience, distress and disturbance of adults interferes tragically with this development, damaging – perhaps permanently – our sense of power, rhythm and timing.

We must remember that there is an innate pleasure in moving our bowels and emptying our bladder when we are ready to. Many adults find this hard to accept, because their own contact with this part of their body has been so much injured. It's a pleasure both of *letting go* and of *pushing out*, which in adult life translates into qualities like groundedness, decisiveness, certainty, balance. The muscles of the pelvis and buttocks are, during the same phase of childhood, learning to ground and balance us as we begin to stand, walk and run.

All of these amazing processes can be wrecked by the effort of massive tension demanded in forcing a too-young child to control their bowels and bladder. The pressure of fear, the desire to please one's parents, push the child into tightening up the whole pelvic floor, the buttocks and thighs, saying 'no' to her own natural functions. Along with this goes the message that her insides, her body contents, are bad and must not be shown to the outside world – the belief, in fact, that she is 'full of shit'.

The messages given by bad toilet training are drastically contradictory, and the child can easily become totally confused. If I poo at one time and place they praise me and tell me how wonderful it is; at a different time and place they shout at me and tell me it's nasty! This gives rise to two simultaneous reactions: that it's my fault and I have to try harder to please everyone, and that it's *their* fault and I hate them.

Remember that small children have a positive, proud attitude towards their poo and wee, an attitude that will later be transferred naturally to other functions, other products of their inner process. But if this possessive pride is attacked by adults' incomprehensible anger, that person may well start to despise herself and all her inner experience; or may become compulsively self-centred, unable to share herself with others. Shame and self-contempt are often part of the holding character which has become stuck around anal issues – and 'stuck' is a particularly apt word here.

Another important factor is likely to be *rage* against adult prohibition and control. The rage itself will be controlled, held in the tight muscles of buttocks and thighs, shoulders and neck – 'my anger is nasty, like shit, and must be contained'. Anger turned inwards often becomes directed at the self in the form of guilt – this is the emotional correlative of physical holding, the person 'feels like shit', like dirt, worthless, foul.

The unsatisfied need, then, is to *let go* and to *push*. It can emerge as adult messiness of all kinds – untidiness, a rushed and confused life style, bad timing, missed appointments. Associated with some of these, there is often a concealed and passive *spitefulness* emanating from the blocked rage, taking the form of letting people down in various ways, failing to meet commitments.

This may be concealed under a thick layer of fawning niceness which is a common feature of the holding character: 'greasy', 'oily', 'arse-licking'. It is as if the holding character is smearing shit all over themselves and us, in an attempt to please which is equally a concealed attack. In this position, we don't expect to be liked. We try hard to appear likeable, with our unreal, constipated smile, but people are not taken in and we end up *being* unlikeable.

The denying holding character manifests in compulsive, rigid, over-controlled attitudes – what we call 'tight-arsed'. The rage has been more or less successfully bound inside as a layer of rigid muscle; the person is being a 'good boy' or a 'good girl', but at a tremendous cost in lost spontaneity and self-regulation. Everything is done by the clock, by the numbers, by the book, by the timetable: 'It's one o'clock, so I must be hungry'. Again, spitefulness can come through in concealed ways, for example the petty bureaucrat who sits heavily on his office potty and finds devious ways of saying 'no'!

A strong holding position often goes along with a heavy, wide body, especially weighty around the shoulders and thighs, and a short neck. There is a tendency for the eyes to retreat into the head within bony, cavernous eye sockets, part of the overall sense of deep suffering often conveyed by the holding character's face. Along with this there is a great strength to endure this suffering, which is composed of desperation, self-hate and hopelessness.

Even a badly stuck holding character will often be very well-grounded; a good, hip-swinging dancer. A successful integration of the themes of holding and control give to the personality a capacity for *effort* which is enjoyable rather than compulsive. Energy can be held and used; there is a quality of determination, patience, taking your time, working *with* the material world rather than against it – a willingness to get your hands dirty.

There is also genuine compassion and service, related to the *fullness* (full heart) of the holding position. Such traits can often be seen, at least in embryo form, in people with anal stuckness – especially the capacity for effort and service. Praising and encouraging these qualities can be very important in developing that crucial, missing sense of self-worth – 'my insides are okay!'

> **Exercise 22**
> Person A sits on a chair, with the whole body constricted and held, head pulled in to the shoulders, and breathing constricted. Focus on the inhale and don't completely breathe out. Breathe into the belly rather than the chest. Person B stands by them and alternates between statements like 'Come on', 'Please', 'There's a lovely boy/girl', etc.; and statements like 'Ugh!' 'That's horrible!' 'How could you!' Again, try to let yourself go into the feelings that come up.

THRUSTING POSITION

Pelvic block against softness: issues of *assertion*

The traditional psychoanalytic name for this position is 'phallic', which comes from the Greek word for penis. In many ways this is seriously misleading, since what is being described is a quality shared equally by girls and boys, though with different effects on the adult character. It arises from the widespread sexist attitude that only those with penises can, or should, thrust.

Once children have developed some sense of holding themselves up and grounding through the buttocks and backs of the legs, they can start literally and symbolically pushing themselves forward. As mobility develops, so does the need for recognition and praise, the desire to assert yourself, to take up space, to show off. Direct sexual exhibitionism is very much part of this: children of four or five are sexual beings, often very hotly so, and need acknowledgement especially from their parents, on whom such feelings will largely be focused. More generally, there is the need to have a say in things, to have some sense of power and autonomy: bedtimes, TV, playing outside are all typical opportunities for assertion.

What so often happens is that adults treat this natural and healthy assertiveness as 'badness', 'wilfulness', 'impudence'. There may even be a conscious intention to crush and overpower the child's will, to frighten it into submission. The classic form of this happens when the father is himself locked into a thrusting position, so that he sees any assertiveness and independence on the part of his children as a threat to his identity, and reacts with physical or emotional violence, the belt or the vicious put-down.

In this situation the child will generally submit – there is little alternative. But built into their character from then on will be a quality of *hatred* and *revenge* that subtly flavours everything they do. A 'yearning thrusting' character will, as an adult, be competitive, pushy, achievement-oriented – a career man or woman.

People who are unable to use their angry energy for worldly success throw their weight around on the domestic, social and sexual fronts instead, or become involved in the machismo of the underworld. Many of these attitudes are strongly encouraged in our culture, primarily in men; thus they are transmitted to the next generation, as a compulsively thrusting and authoritarian parent represses their child's independence and sets them up for the same script.

The ability to push and thrust with the pelvis – in a soft and feeling way – is essential to satisfying sex for both women and men; and the corresponding life capacity is equally important. In the thrusting-block character position, there is an overlay of hate and fear in such pelvic movement, a fear of *collapse* (in the face of adult power), leading to an attitude which Reich called 'genital revenge'. If the person is a man, then they may be a rapist, overt or indirect; if a woman, what men call a 'ballbreaker', using sex to humiliate (though men often use this label to attack any woman who scares them with her healthy sexual assertiveness). The soft easy thrust becomes a violent harsh movement – 'screwing'.

Sexually speaking, the yearning thruster will be a Don Juan character who uses sex to 'score' – for conquest and ego satisfaction rather than pleasure and melting contact. Similar attitudes will colour their attitude to life in general – enjoyment takes second place to status. Our culture tends actively to encourage such distortions in men, to the extent of seeing them as intrinsically manly, macho, butch. A woman or girl who shows such traits will often be met with disapproval and invalidation ('tomboy', 'unfeminine') even though the thrusting may be entirely healthy, the natural urge for assertiveness and achievement.

The body type that goes with the thrusting character is quite highly rated in our society: it tends to be large, well-muscled, energetic, athletic – at any rate in milder versions of the block. The stronger the block, the more the body tends to be rigid, musclebound and overcharged. Someone who *denies* their need to thrust will necessarily have a rigid body and character, often sex-negative, self-righteous and moralistic. This is a different strategy for genital revenge – 'stamp out this menace!' The absence of pleasure is even clearer with these compulsively 'good' people. Thrusting characters often suffer from 'stress-related ailments', because they put themselves through so much stress.

The creative side of the thrusting character is its energy, drive, courage, ambition, physical and mental élan; its willpower and discipline. The distortions stem from insecurity, from the fear of being smashed down which is hidden under an exaggerated 'strength', able to brook no equals, let alone 'superiors'. In its obsession with rank, pecking order, competition, and in its assumption that every situation must involve a winner and loser, the thrusting block is clearly a central factor in patriarchal society.

> **Exercise 23**
> Person B stands on a chair; person A stands looking up at them, legs braced stiffly, jaw stuck out, chest stuck out, fists clenched. Use your breath to puff yourself up. A says things like 'No', 'I won't'; B says 'Oh yes you will', 'You better had', 'Do what I tell you', etc. After a while, make contact and reverse.

CRISIS POSITION

Pelvic block against opening: issues of *contact*

This is what psychoanalysts call the 'hysteric' character; just as 'phallic' comes from the Greek for penis, 'hysteric' comes from the Greek for womb. Again this represents a *social* reality, for in our culture there is much more scope and acceptance for women in the crisis position than there is for men. All children however, boys as much as girls, have to confront the issues around pelvic opening, which arise when self-assertion begins to encounter the reality of another person, and of the social world.

    A fundamental fact about human beings is that they have gender. In our society, gender has a very particular set of *meanings* attached to it. Saying that someone is a man or a woman, a girl or a boy, is doing much more than stating what is between their legs. It establishes a whole set of expectations about their appearance, their range of movements and sounds, their activities, their attitudes, their personality, their 'nature' – it is not too huge a simplification to say that our society splits the range of human behaviour into two halves, allowing one half to males and the other half to females.

    We can't go into the possible reasons for this process here, beyond pointing out that most societies, perhaps all, do something like this, though they often give very different *contents* to the male and female halves. From the point of view of a small child, coming face to face with this reality for the first time, its implications are disastrous.

    A little girl, even today, is asked to accept that she is cut off from the world of power and freedom offered to her brother – and usually represented by the father. A little boy is asked to accept that he is cut off from the world of warmth and softness usually represented by the mother (an important way in which this is expressed is that he 'can't have babies'). Each is presented with huge deprivations and huge compensations, but the whole issue is handled indirectly and inexplicitly, and is coloured by adults' own, often unconscious, distress about gender.

The issue is also tied up, both developmentally and by its nature, with that of opening up to loving and pleasurable contact with other human beings. The self-asserting little child focuses its erotic energy on the close adults around, usually its parents. (We are using 'it' instead of 'her' in this section to avoid the conventional association of the crisis character with being female.) The parents themselves have succumbed to gender roles, and are openly or unconsciously telling the child to conform. They do this at the same time as, and partly *through*, openly or unconsciously reacting to the child's intense sexual energy, either pushing it away or encouraging it – often both at once!

One powerful way of describing all this is to use Freud's term, the 'Oedipus Complex'. This focuses on the issues of power, possession and jealousy in the classic nuclear family. It describes very real events, though in a way that does not sufficiently question gender stereotyping or bring out the underlying issues of social conformity. This is the point at which the child is about to emerge into the social world; its acceptance of gender conventions, and all the subtle seductions and abuses that they imply, is the price of entry.

It's no surprise that a child faced with these vast ramifications, with this elaborate combination of carrot and big stick, will generally react with some degree of panic. The core of this will be what we can describe as 'biological' panic, a response to the opening-up of energy that accompanies the 'first puberty' at around five or six. This involves an increase in charge, similar to that of the teenage 'second puberty', of which anyone will be aware who spends time with open eyes around young children.

Surrender to pleasure, to the streaming of energy in our bodies, is for almost all of us accompanied by anxiety and fear. We want to open, yet are desperately scared to. Instead we react with some version of freezing or exploding, fighting or fleeing, under- or overactivity; with a frantically erotic style of being (the yearning block) or with retreat, denial of sexual feeling altogether.

For a very large number of children, this natural response gets very much amplified by the interference of *adult* sexuality. The innocent erotic energy of children at this age can produce sexual excitement in a lot of grown-ups whose own sexual development has been damaged. We now have some idea just how many children have been sexually abused by adults, often during this first puberty but sometimes much earlier. The natural anxiety of opening-up then becomes a fully fledged panic, as the child is forced to deal with experiences that are wholly inappropriate for them.

This adult invasion can take very subtle forms as well: it is often an atmosphere of flirting and seductiveness, rather than any overt physical act. Alternatively, adults can react to their own arousal by blaming the child and suppressing the child's sexuality. The child knows in its bodymind what is going on, but has no way of verbalising it even to itself. Both physical and emotional interference plug into the general sexual violence of the situation – the child is being pressurised in many ways to fit his or her erotic energy into the straitjacket of socially accepted gender roles.

The 'crisis character' is a component in all of us, though usually stronger in those who have had to deal with a heavier dose of sexual abuse, physical or emotional (the holding and boundary positions seem the other response to abuse). As we have said, its main tactics are freezing or exploding – opposite ways of trying to flee an intolerable excitement.

These responses generally get submerged in children. After the flurry of sexual charge and interest at about five, six or seven, they enter a 'latent phase' of apparent asexuality (in our culture at least) until puberty recurs in the form of physical sexual maturity. But the sexual attitudes which then emerge are essentially *re*-emerging: they were formed during the 'first puberty', on the basis of how the child's already existing character armour confronted the issue of pelvic opening in the context of adult sexual pressure.

In adults, the crisis position tends to sexualise every issue because it is tied to a development phase which is itself sexual. The process is often unconscious, but it can be very obvious to other people as a sort of continual seductiveness in the person's behaviour and body language, or conversely as an 'uprightness', an extraordinary heightened sensitivity to sexual implications which makes one scared of offending them with quite innocent remarks. Both attitudes can even appear in the same person at the same time.

It's clear that these are attitudes traditionally validated in women, either separately or in combination: the virgin and the vamp. They mask panic, and represent an inability to surrender to deep sexual feelings for fear of being overwhelmed and losing control (which may literally have happened in childhood abuse). At the same time, there is a strong *need* for sexual contact, so there is often a teasing, flirting tone, not necessarily conscious – an exaggeration of healthy playfulness, 'sexiness', foreplay, dressing up, dancing – all sorts of creative and enjoyable behaviour which is 'sexy but not sex'. What's missing is relaxation and commitment: the opening block sets up a constant yes/no/yes/no pattern, again traditionally seen as 'feminine'.

But men are as likely as women to occupy the crisis position – perhaps more often in a pseudo-thrusting form. The yearning version will thus be an ersatz macho posturing, all leather and heavy metal, while the denying form might be hysterical puritanism. Until recently, and still in many communities, the only socially viable way for men to express the full crisis character was in the gay subculture.

What makes the crisis position recognisable is its air of panic, of high charge. Everything is life or death. There is often either a theatrical exaggeration to the person's style, or a deathly stillness which is equally theatrical. The body type that develops with a strong crisis position is less clearly defined than in some other cases, but in one way or another it tends to give a strongly sexual impression, which may be attractive or repulsive – or both – to other people. Crisis characters often stir people up, this being their unconscious intention as a way of sharing the panic around, camouflaging their own terror and excitement.

We can think of the energy in a crisis character shooting around the body looking for some other lodging apart from the genitals; any other form of excitement is preferable, safer. So the crisis character mimics all the other character positions – which can be very confusing for therapists! In particular, someone deeply involved in the crisis position often comes over at first as a vulnerable, 'schiz-y' boundary character. In fact crisis characters are quite tough, though they may not feel it. There is a special relationship between these two extremes of the character range, of head and tail, and energy can swing powerfully between them.

The underlying strength and resilience often gives people the idea that a crisis character is 'pretending', could 'pull themselves together if they just made an effort'. In a sense they are pretending, but the pretence is an *involuntary* reaction to deep panic. The panic is completely rational in origin: dangerous and scary things *did* happen. Freud worked with extreme crisis characters who experienced 'hysterical paralysis' with no physical causation: a pretence in one sense, but outside any willed control or awareness. Often, though, the game playing is both conscious and unconscious: panic and anxiety fog the ability to look coolly at what one is really doing. It can be amazing how a crisis character in a state of chaos can 'snap out of it' when asked.

Yet crisis characters can play games for very high stakes. Living permanently on their nerves and by their wits, out on the edge, they develop a strange sort of coolness. Like combat veterans, someone constantly in the crisis position learns to live with terror. It is likely that almost everyone who works in a directly life-threatening occupation is either a thrusting character, testing and proving themselves, or a crisis character fuelled by their own panic.

It is when we are occupying the crisis position that we tend to create *bodily* expressions of our conflicts: the well-known 'hysterical symptoms' which mimic physical illness to act out an emotional state. Yet is there a real distinction? More and more we see all physical illnesses as the expression of a conflict, a life crisis which is potentially healing. Perhaps crisis characters, with their penchant for melodrama and staginess, are simply the ones who get caught at it – accidentally on purpose!

There are many attractive and creative features in the crisis character. Perhaps the most obvious is their sexiness, but more generally there is their fun and excitement, the lively energy and 'game-for-anything' attitude, together with their subtle and perceptive understanding of roles and rules (the better to break them). These qualities contribute a great deal of spice to life.

Perhaps the greatest contribution of the crisis attitude in us all is its *refusal of patriarchy*, and of the gender roles forced on us. Crisis characters may find some weird and exotic modes of rebellion, but rebel they do! At root, what they are demanding is very simple: the right to choose. To choose what sort of sexual contact they have; to choose to be playful and childlike, not always urgent and direct; above all, to choose not to be abused.

> **Exercise 24**
> This is the hardest position to act out, but try the following: A stands still, breathing into their pelvis with the emphasis on breathing out, while B alternates between trying to attract them – 'Come here', 'I want you', 'Aren't you sweet' etc. – and rejecting them once they respond: 'No, no', 'Not like that', 'Come on, that's enough'. A, try to let your whole body really respond to each message; B, let yourself be fully seductive, and then switch into complete coldness. After a while, make contact with each other before you switch roles.

OPEN POSITION?

No permanent blocks: issue of *surrender*

In the first edition of this book, following Reich (who called it the 'genital character'), we had a section here about the 'open character', which we described as 'a true acceptance of reality and pleasure, a surrender to their own nature and to that larger Nature of which we are part'. We still believe in the reality and importance of that *experience*; but we no longer want to describe it as a 'character position' alongside the others we have been discussing.

Identifying a 'healthy' character tends to encourage a negative view of the rest, as pieces of pathology, ways of being not OK. Increasingly we have come to believe that every character position contributes important creative qualities to being human. In order to be here as embodied beings, we each have to be *someone*, to have certain preferences, certain concerns, certain styles. Ultimately, this is all that character is: a particular flavour or colour of being human.

However, the more traumatic our experience of particular growth thresholds has been, the more narrow and circumscribed our behaviour is likely to be – the more we can also get stuck in a groove, fixated on one particular aspect of life to the exclusion of all others, trying to open every door we encounter with the same key – or perhaps, if our early experience has been unlucky, with a bit of broken metal that we *think* is a key. Character can function as a container for the light, or as a means of hiding it. Usually, it has some of each quality.

The key quality, then, is flexibility – openness to reality and the ways in which it shifts and changes. No one is permanently without blocks: armouring appears in reaction to events, and can disappear again as the individual breathes, lets go, cries or laughs or yells or yawns, struggles or accepts – and moves on.

At our most open – as distinct from an open *position*, which itself sounds like a fixed and rigid way of being – we have access to the full range of powers and capacities appropriate to each character position described above. We manifest these qualities creatively; we can see, think, feel, enjoy, relate, lead, hold on, take our time, assert, reach out, play and open up, because we are secure in our right to exist, to be received, to be validated, to value ourselves, thrust ourselves forward, and choose the contact we have with others. We have the right and the ability to be fully human.

7

More on Character

> Perhaps all the dragons of our lives are princesses who are only waiting to see us once beautiful and brave.
>
> Rainer Maria Rilke, *Letters to a Young Poet*

> He who fights too long against dragons becomes a dragon himself.
>
> Nietzsche, *On the Geneology of Morals*

You may have found the last chapter both too complicated and too simplistic; and it is simplified, in the sense that 'nobody is really like that' – it's not possible to reduce a real person to the cardboard categories of the character positions. We can recognise strong elements of an individual's nature, but there is always a 'yes, but', some other strand or tendency which makes the picture richer and more complex.

In this chapter we want to show how we can flesh out the bones, and use the concepts of character to generate something more like real human beings. Looked at another way, it means that we can use these concepts to understand real human beings. First, though, to help with the complexity of the material and the ramification of confusing detail, here is a summary of the character positions described so far, together with a selection of keywords for each position.

A SUMMARY OF THE CHARACTER POSITIONS

Boundary position
(womb, birth and first weeks)

> Eye segment block. Theme of existence: the right to be
> *Stuck:* fragility – invasion – unreality
> *Creative:* Perceptive – inspired – psychic
> *Keywords:* Distant ... Blank ... Deep ... Vulnerable ... Foggy ... In pieces ... Cold ... Crazy ... Scary ... Weird ... Bizarre ... Paranoid ... Keep off! ...

Oral position
(feeding, weaning, siblings)

Jaw and mouth block. Theme of need: the right to be fed and supported
Stuck: Unfair world – misunderstood – hungry – empty
Creative: Appetite for life – nurturing – eloquent
Keywords: Needy ... Exhausting ... Draining ... Love-starved ... Manipulative ... Persuasive ... Biting ... Sharp-tongued ... Greedy ... Ungrounded ... Sulky ... Arrogant ... Clever ... Tired ... Won't ... Black ...

Control position
(beginning independence, using adults as play objects)

Chest segment block. Theme of validation: the right to have my experience acknowledged
Stuck: No one else is real – need to dominate, to get my way, or else to hide
Creative: Big hearted – leadership – looking after
Keywords: Dominant ... Overwhelming ... Seductive ... Bossy ... Charismatic ... Top dog ... How to Win Friends and Influence People ,,, Puffed-up ... Insincere ... Impressive ... Hard sell ... Cut-off ... Politico ... Hail-Fellow-Well-Met ... Unreal ...

Holding position
(toilet training, timetabling, pressure to 'behave')

Anal block, buttocks, thighs, shoulders. Theme of control: the right to value myself, to take my time
Stuck: Self-disgust – repression – suffering
Creative: Grounded – patient – determined – compassionate
Keywords: Long-suffering ... Painful ... Tortured ... Enduring ... Held-in ... Stuck ... Bursting ... Sturdy ... Guilty ... Full of shit ... Arse-licking ... Greasy ... Oily ... Sticky ... Repulsive ... Bully, petty tyrant ... Obsessive ... Repetitive ... Maddening ...

Thrusting position
(rebellion, independence, punishment)

Pelvic block against softness. Theme of assertion: the right to take up space, be noticed
Stuck: Competition – revenge – mustn't collapse
Creative: Initiative – courage – physicality
Keywords: Pushy ... Proud ... Competitive ... Abrasive ... Macho ... Rigid ... Effective ... Overpowering ... Athletic ...

Upright ... Golden girl/boy ... Egotistical ... Keeping their act together ... Driving ... Driven ... Exhibitionist ...

Crisis position
(entering the social world, taking on gender)

Pelvic block against surrender. Theme of contact: the right to choose, to play, to be ambiguous
Stuck: Sexual panic – yes/no – confusion – melodrama
Creative: Playful – graceful – complex – exciting
Keywords: Jumpy ... Over-the-top ... Dramatic ... Exciting ... Sexual ... Flirty ... Stirring ... Attractive ... Frustrating ... Confusing ... Evasive/Elusive ... Frozen ... Scared ... Boundary (often first impression) ...

Our idea in using these keywords is not that each one applies to every person manifesting that character position. We are aiming more at a 'splatter effect', since we find in practice that if we want to use *several* terms from one section about a given individual (or other equivalent words), then that person will be strongly involved with the corresponding character position.

So, for example, if I find myself thinking how *pushy*, *proud* and *rigid* a new client is, then I will realise that they have a strong *thrusting* component in their makeup. If I find myself seeing them as *needy*, *negative* and *exhausting*, then I am tuning in to their *oral* material. Or if I experience them as *clever*, *persuasive* and *arrogant,* I am meeting a different sort of oral character, and so on.

Clearly, some of the keywords in each section point in very different directions, or even contradict each other. A given character position can express itself in very different ways: for example, as either a 'yearning' or a 'denying' attitude. Similarly, one keyword on its own might fit with several different character positions; for example, above we have used 'proud' for a thrusting character and 'arrogant' for an oral character. It is the appropriateness of *several* keywords from one section that gives us useful information.

You will perhaps have noticed that many, though not all, of the keywords have negative connotations. As we will explain at more length in Chapter 8, it is often through our negative reactions to clients that we can learn most about their character. But it is important to stress that no judgement is intended. These are the emotional reactions that the unhealthy aspects of character structure tend to bring up, particularly in the intense atmosphere of the therapy session but also in everyday interactions. They are not, however, assessments of a person's worth.

As well as being differentiated through the yearning or denying attitude involved, each character position is very much affected by what is going on in the rest of the person besides the segment directly concerned. In this context a human being is rather like a hologram, where each part both reflects the whole and is reflected in the whole.

Let's take as an example the holding character position. As we have seen, this position derives from blocking in the pelvis, especially the anus, buttocks and thighs; this blocking becomes a general attitude of holding on, influencing the overall shape of the body (wide and heavy), and creating a tendency to some specific physical traits like heavy shoulders, short neck, sunken eyes and so on. Together with this goes the overall issue of self-disgust and self-control, letting go and holding on.

This overall holding position may be combined with blocking in any of the other segments, both those at 'top and tail' – which we have seen as defining the character positions – and in the other 'central' segments – neck, heart, waist and belly. So the basic themes and attitudes will take on different forms and express themselves through different issues, like a beam of light shone through different coloured filters.

A helpful way of looking at this with the holding position is that in each segment there will be either an attempt to *hold on* (denying version) or an attempt to *let go* (yearning version), manifested through the physical and emotional repertoire *of that segment*.

Thus a holding character with an eye block will either be trying to *let go through the eyes and mind*, or trying to *hold on through the eyes and mind*. The issue of boundaries, fragmentation and containment will be there, but as a way of approaching these issues of holding on and letting go. Holding on with the eye segment, then, might result in the development of complex intellectual systems, even obsessions; elaborate, essentially pointless thought processes which are really a sort of 'mental constipation', never reaching the point. A yearning version, concerned with letting go, might either be mentally 'messy' and chaotic, or else applying the same sort of systematic order to meditation techniques.

A holding character with an oral block tends to show the anal material through the mouth, either as a denying style of tight lips, pinched nostrils and general disgust, as if other people leave a bad taste or smell, or as a yearning version which uses the mouth to spread shit around, a sticky, greasy, oily, 'arse-licking' character disguising an underlying spiteful malice.

The same principle applies to any combination of blocks with any basic character. A thrusting character with a neck block will be 'stiff-necked', rigid, refusing to bow down to anyone – and as a result refusing any softness and givingness, 'holier-than-thou'. An oral character with an eye block will have issues about being 'fed' through their eyes, and will display either a 'Teach me O Master' passivity (yearning version) or a stubborn refusal to be shown, taught or met (denying version). And so on.

Thus we can build up the uniqueness of an individual character structure through the combination of different blocks in the bodymind, and read the 'story' which that combination tells. It would be pointless, and endless, to try to list every possible combination – like illustrating every possible fingerprint – but the table summarises the meetings of pairs of different character positions, each of which will in practice be influenced by various degrees and kinds of blocking in all the *other* segments. What is more meaningful, of course, is working in the opposite direction, recognising what blocks and issues are operating in real people.

It may seem impossible for any real use to be made of this great mass of material – as soon as it stops being simplistic, it becomes unmanageable! In practice, though, we get immense help from the system of character analysis; not so much on the level of intellectual understanding as through a developing capacity to recognise character attitudes on a gut level. Much of what we are saying about character is embedded in the folk wisdom of our language itself, with all its body imagery: 'stiff necked', 'feet on the ground', 'arse-licker', 'pushy', 'cold-hearted'. All these terms are direct pointers to the essence of someone's character structure. Now we turn towards what we can call the 'bridge' character positions that seem to arise so frequently. These manifest when a person seems to exist mainly between two character positions which are adjacent in terms of the sequence of energy from boundary to crisis: between holding and crisis, for example, or between boundary and oral; either oscillating between the two according to circumstances, or else firmly straddling the divide and combining elements of each into a personal synthesis.

BOUNDARY/ORAL BRIDGE

This is the common intellectual character position: trying to make words and ideas into a self-sufficient reality – using them as nourishment, as protection, as contact, as erotic play, as a substitute for the life of the *body* self-contained within the *head*. There is often an important seat of tension at the physical junction between the two segments, the soft palate and the internal cavity of the head; there can be a sense of a 'watcher' inside the head, unable to let go into the sensuous life of the body through fear of being overwhelmed.

Conversely, a valuable quality of this intellectual position is its resistance to being overwhelmed by feeling, and by the pressure of other people's presence.

ORAL/CONTROL BRIDGE

Someone in this position is going to find it impossible to express any needs they may have. They may end up indirectly acting out their needs by taking care of other people – treating them as small and weak, whether they are or not, because that is how they feel themselves inside. But there will be a bossy, 'for-your-own-good' quality to the supposed caring which will generally alienate its recipients. Some social workers, politicians and therapists are acting from this part of themselves.

CONTROL/HOLDING BRIDGE

Here the jammed-up, stuck, inflated side of each of these positions is emphasised, and the individual may have a very off-putting 'constipated' quality to them. Rather than controlling themselves in the holding style, they may try to control *other people*, expressing punitive, moralistic and repressive attitudes. Here we find the classic bureaucrat who secretly loves sitting on everyone else's freedom and initiative. But also, instead of letting go themselves, they may try to force other people to let go, in a style of repressive liberalism or radicalism. 'PC' behaviour can be used as a channel for this sort of attitude.

In the background of the control/holding bridge there is always a little girl or boy trying desperately, but hopelessly, to be *good:* good enough to be acceptable. In their drive for goodness they may lay waste to whole families or communities.

HOLDING/THRUSTING BRIDGE

This produces the ultimate *rigid* character, binding all their energy into tense musculature and fixed attitudes: a combination of the holder's terror of opening up, and the thruster's terror of collapse. People in this position often have very strict moral codes and strong consciences, blaming themselves heavily for any slight lapse from grace. There is often an underlying fantasy of shitting themselves, becoming 'soiled', 'disgraced', as if their insides will fall out and be lost forever if they let go of their control. There will be deep tension within the pelvis, and usually also in the back muscles. Such people very often take out their tension on others, becoming moral arbiters and censors; at source their hateful anger is directed at the people who suppressed their own natural vitality and pleasure.

92 Reichian Growth Work

BOUNDARY	ORAL	CONTROL
Y Seeking release from panic through the head. Wild ideas, crazy visions. Flirting. / Blank, confused. Pseudo-schizophrenic states. 'Playing crazy'. D	Y Seeking release from panic through the mouth. Overeating, overtalking, substance abuse / Lost, depressed, 'can't explain'. Eating disorders. D	Y Seeking release from panic through controlling others. Seductive, vamp, charismatic. / 'Follow me and stamp out sex' D
Y Peering, narrow-eyed, suspicious of attack - 'paranoid'. / Obsessive, blinkered, persecuting, litigious. D	Y 'I must succeed but can't succeed'; bipolar, addictive. / 'It's hopeless, I'm useless, no good' taking comfort from food, substance abuse. D	Y Crusader, gangbuster, populist politico, team captain. / Gangster, generalissimo, political boss. D
Y Trying to let go with the eyes/mind - e.g. through enlightenment systems / Trying to hold on with the eyes/mind - e.g. through intellectual and philosophical systems D	Y Fawningly polite, 'oily', 'greasy' - hidden spite 'Shit-eater'. / Tight-lipped, puritanical, smugly superior. D	Y 'I will force you to express yourself' (Reich!) 'You must admire my shit' (self-expression) / Tightly controlling of others. 'You must admire my self-discipline'. D
Y Seeking recognition through eyes/mind - e.g. inspirational teacher. / Seeking control through eyes/mind - e.g. guru, hypnotist. D	Y Using eloquence and charm to control others and get needs met while concealing them. / 'I have no needs or feelings; I control you by taking care of you'. D	Y 'I pretend to be loveable in order to get your attention.' / 'I get your attention through dominating or manipulating you.' D
Y Seeking to be fed through the eyes/mind - e.g. disciple. / Words and ideas used as a defense against being seen. D	Y Needy, complaining, dependent, sometimes endearing. / 'I have no needs - I can do it all myself'. D	ORAL
Y Need to see/understand so as to feel real; underbounded, lost. / Taking refuge in thought and fantasy to escape the dangers of real life. D	BOUNDARY	

More on Character

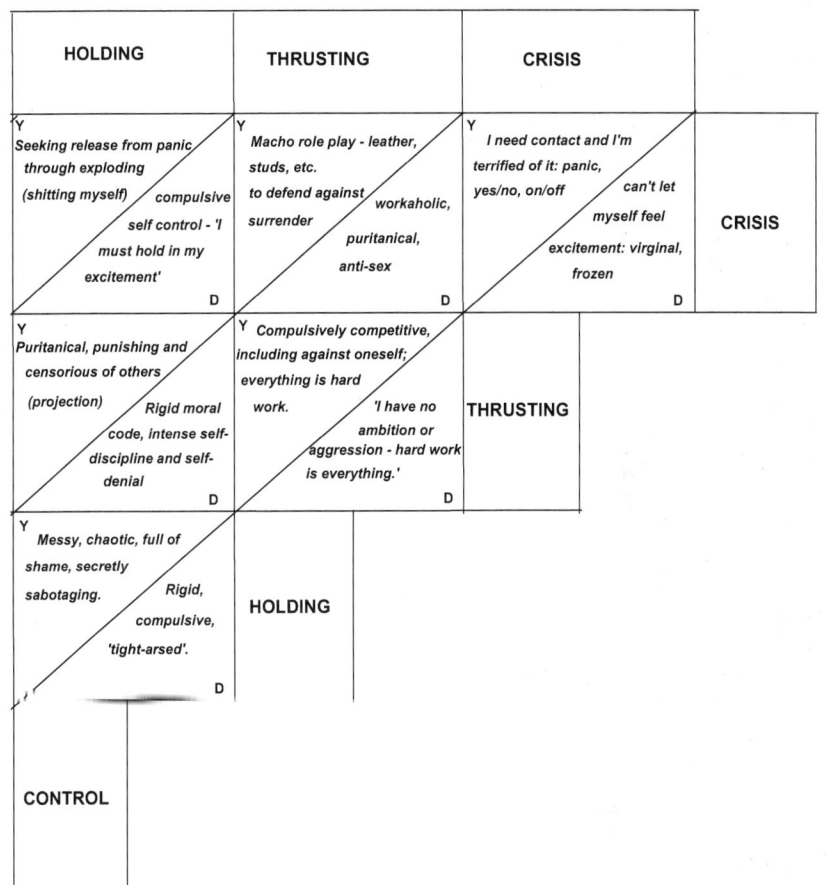

CHARACTER COMBINATIONS

The longest diagonal, towards the right of the chart, shows the basic character positions; other boxes show how blocks in more than one segment might influence each other. These are suggestions only - there are other possibilities.

Y = yearning version; D = denying version

HOLDING/CRISIS BRIDGE

These are not strictly 'adjacent' positions according to our system, but the bridge between them seems to be a very common one. It is specifically about flight from the *thrusting* position which would come between the two. If someone is deeply unwilling or unable to occupy the thrusting position and assert themselves in a solidly committed way, they often tend to oscillate between the excitement and movement of the crisis character, and a collapse into holding self-dislike and stuckness. It's a sort of 'manic-depressive' pattern, moving from an exaggerated sense of power and charisma into a morning-after feeling of 'Oh God, what have I done, what must people think of me?'

We often find a strong diaphragm block associated with this position, giving a breathless jerkiness to the person's self-expression. The block derives from panic about self-assertion, perhaps because of scary authoritarian parenting.

THRUSTING/CRISIS BRIDGE

This is a particularly difficult combination to sustain, since the two positions are in many ways chalk and cheese. Any expression of traditionally 'masculine' attitudes which feels *hollow* (both in men and women), a performance rather than a reality, is probably to do with this bridge position: the parodic pseudo-machismo of some gay men's circles, for instance, or men who feel pushed to act in violent or otherwise extreme ways to 'defend' their masculinity. This is the position which classical psychoanalysis talks about in terms of 'repressed homosexuality', but what is really being repressed is openness and contact, understood in patriarchal terms as unmasculine. There is a flight from softness into a pretence of toughness. People in this position confront in their own bodies the *political* problem of combining power and tenderness in a patriarchal society. The focus of tension in the body can be the perineum, the area between anus and genitals.

CRISIS/BOUNDARY BRIDGE

Although these two positions are at opposite ends of the cycle, they are also closely linked: Alexander Lowen has pointed out a tendency for energy to swing between the two. Both positions are based on *panic*. For the crisis character it is panic about contact, and for the boundary character about existence, but it is easy to see how each theme can feed into the other. The leading characteristic of someone occupying this bridge position will be chaos, together with a deep elusiveness: they are almost impossible to pin down, which is as frustrating for them as it is for anyone else!

Let's move away now from this precision and detail and get back in touch with the main issue of character: that it embodies *at the same time* our attempts to engage with existence, and our attempts to run away from it.

The 'energy-exchange segments' are our most important channels of contact with the world, including other people. Each of these segments, through the nature of the organ systems and subtle energy channels involved and because of the phase of life during which our energy is focused there, takes on a particular 'flavour', an innate style of being. All these flavours blend to make up a whole human being, able to relate to the world in a rich, complex and flexible way.

At the same time each segment, each channel, throws up its own problems and challenges; sets up the potential for fixation, for blocking – again, in the particular style and flavour of the segment concerned. Yet neither our 'failure' nor our 'success' in negotiating the challenges of a particular phase is going to be total; there is always a mixture, a balance of more or less free or bound energy, which establishes the terms of a person's relationship with this particular aspect of existence. This balance is constantly shifting as the circumstances of our lives put more or less pressure on our capacity to cope.

Then there is the mixture and balance of each segment with every other segment, creating a complex unity which expresses that person's unique style of being in the world. The first thing to do, always, with this unique character structure is to *celebrate* it, as a brilliantly successful strategy for surviving a threatening environment.

If we then start to help someone question their strategy, highlighting ways in which it limits their potential for growth and pleasure, this is not to belittle the achievement, or the often astonishing beauty and strength of that human being. Character is a way of growing in safety. Therapy exists only to support and to *extend* that capacity for growth – not to undermine what someone has already created in herself.

It remains true, though, and must emerge clearly from all that we have said in the last two chapters about the individual character positions, that character is also a way of *not* growing. It is a brilliant way of surviving an environment which is, let us face it, appalling. The deforming influence of capitalism and patriarchy corrupts even the best and most loving family, so that the strength and beauty we display as adults is like the strength and beauty of a Japanese bonsai tree: essentially a stunted caricature of what a healthy full-grown specimen would be.

8

Therapy

> Be strong then, and enter into your own body;
> there you have a solid place for your feet.
> Think about it carefully!
> Don't go off somewhere else!
>
> Kabir says this: just throw away all thoughts of imaginary things, and stand firm in that which you are.
>
> Robert Bly, *The Kabir Book*

So what can we do about all this? About the tension and defensiveness, the illusions and pretences, the inability to face life and pleasure? The ideas about people that we have outlined have not been plucked out of thin air; they have developed through the experience of giving and receiving therapy, and in turn they have led to new therapeutic approaches.

This book is not a *'How to ...'* manual. Reichian therapy can't be learnt out of books, and some of its detailed techniques could be misunderstood or mishandled by someone who had only read about them and never seen them in action. This is not to say that everyone has to rely on specialised experts with elite knowledge. There is very definitely a role for self-help, for peer therapy sessions exchanged between ordinary people, and a part of our work is teaching people how to do this. But such teaching, we feel, has to happen face to face and heart to heart. What we can do here is describe the background to the practice of therapy, and also communicate some of the flavour of the experience.

There is a central emphasis in Reichian work on *contact:* contact between client and therapist, contact between the client and her own inner life. As therapists, we are in a sense always offering ourselves to the other person – offering our attention, our aliveness, our heart: always working to clear away the blocks on both sides against heart-to-heart connection. We are coming from our own core, that central place of love and wholesomeness we described in Chapter

6; trying to reach the core of the other person, their essential, undamaged health.

This necessarily means that each therapist works in their own style, expressing their own nature. And this style has to adapt itself in response to each client, meeting them in a way which is appropriate for *this* person at *this* moment. The wholeness of an individual can be expressed as energy, as thought, as emotion, as body, and it may be right to meet them on any of these levels in a given situation, depending on where they 'live' within their self, which of these channels they are able to experience.

This does not mean that we always work with a person's preferred channel, of course! A 'thinker' may be challenged to feel, a 'body' to connect with life energy which is not simply physical, and so on. But the emphasis is on finding contact, which means starting from what *is*, from the points of openness and closedness in the relationship which begin to manifest as soon as two people are together.

Let's look in turn at how our therapy operates in each of these four spheres: body, emotion, thought and energy, remembering that the distinction is somewhat artificial, but also a useful way of bringing out the essence of the therapeutic relationship.

BODY

Many people who have heard of Reichian therapy think of it primarily as 'bodywork'. Reich was certainly the first psychotherapist in modern times to focus primarily on the body, reminding us that this is where and how we live. Most Reichians are strongly oriented towards breathing, muscle tension, posture and touch; but we are not primarily trying to 'correct' someone's armouring, as for instance a remedial massage practitioner might do. Our bodywork is aimed essentially at awakening the life energy in the body, trusting that once awake it will know what to do, how to heal.

So we encourage our clients to breathe, not according to an ideal pattern, but simply to breathe more deeply, more freely, with less control than they are used to – to 'let breathing breathe'. People's customary style of breathing varies enormously: what for one individual would be a deep breath may for another be normal, or even shallow. Similarly, different people tend to breathe with different parts of their body – you may see one person's belly rise and sink with the breath while their chest stays almost motionless; the next person may expand and contract their chest without moving their belly at all.

> **Exercise 25**
> Try this with a few friends: let each person in turn lie on their back and breathe, without trying to influence their breath at all. Look for the differences in depth; in comparative strength of inbreath and outbreath; in which parts of the body move with the breathing. You may be amazed by how variously we perform this most basic of activities! Remember that this is an exploration, not a competition: take the opportunity to simply perceive and be with the other person's breath, witnessing without judgement.

We start from where each person is, encouraging them to bring their awareness to their breath and see what it wants to do. Whatever form of work we are doing, part of our attention will be on the client's breathing, but for bodywork as such we generally ask them to lie on their back on a mattress while we sit or kneel beside them. (Before we engage in this way we will have spent some time, often several sessions, building up a relationship between us.)

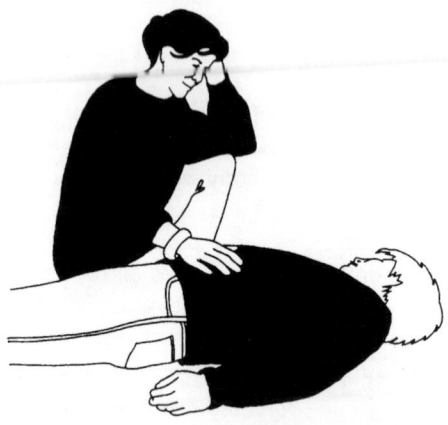

Then we watch, in contact with our own breath and our own naturalness, which is the only way to encourage it to manifest in another person. After a while we perhaps start to ask the client, if they are not already telling us, what they notice about their own breathing; and to feed back what we see, to point out where the breath moves and where it doesn't, how one person, for instance, breathes *in* more strongly and *out* more weakly, or vice versa; how someone moves their lungs only from half empty to completely empty and back again, never really letting them fill up; how another person never really lets their lungs empty; how someone's outbreath catches in their throat rather than sighing out freely. Through this dialogue we try to help the client to become aware of what they do, and if this feels right, to relax a little way into a fuller, freer breath; alternatively, they may explore the limitation and tension in their breath.

In a while, we may perhaps put our hands on the person's chest and belly, encouraging the outbreath to deepen by leaning gently into them, then taking our weight back as the breath returns. We might rock their body from side to side, or massage the chest and shoulders, all as part of inviting a relaxed, easy but strong breathing to develop while at the same time offering the implicit reassurance and challenge of physical touch.

For many people, a few minutes' conscious focus on their breath is in itself enough to create powerful new sensations and emotions, as the stronger breath puts a stronger charge into their body. If we are loose and relaxed to start with, the experience can be pleasant, empowering – even ecstatic. If there is a fair amount of tension, though, more difficult and perhaps alarming feelings appear as new energy hits the muscle blocks.

The emotions that have been 'held' in the muscle armour use the breath energy to push for expression, while at the same time the blocks themselves are taking up some of the new energy in order to push back. The whole contradiction which armouring embodies, between expression and repression, is intensified, which can be very uncomfortable both physically and emotionally.

Thus the client will need careful support through this part of the process. Above all, they need to know that someone is there with them, and that what is happening is basically OK. We will also encourage them to let movement happen wherever there is a sense of stuck energy; to express that charge, maybe by stretching, wriggling around on the mattress, hitting out at the mattress with hands or feet, screwing up or opening wide the eyes, bouncing with the pelvis. Often it's a matter of noticing and amplifying the slight movements that are already happening. At the same time, we remind them to *keep breathing* and to *make a sound*.

The voice is very powerful, perhaps essential, for the release of held tension. It focuses our awareness like a spotlight on the area of the body where we are working. It encourages us to breathe and to 'push'; and, of course, it also directly expresses the held emotion.

Often the person isn't immediately in touch with the feeling that is being held in. If we persuade them to make a sound, it will start as a flat, toneless 'Aaaaaaa', then begin to take on emotional colouring. Without making any conscious effort it may become a yell of anger, a scream of fear, a cry of pain or grief – even a roar of laughter or a shout of affirmation. Once this point of connection with and commitment to a feeling has been reached, the whole sense of stuck tension in the body suddenly turns over. The energy has peaked in this act of expression and remembering – the bodymind has become whole again. As the storm passes there will generally be a sense of release, relaxation and spaciousness.

How easily such a point can be reached depends on the extent and the nature of the body armouring. Sometimes, breathing *without* bodily expression of feeling will create a situation of extreme held tension. The person will start to feel a stiffness and uncomfortable tingling in certain areas, often the hands and around the mouth, and will find it hard to *stop* breathing deeply – a state which, if left to take its course, would gradually become both excruciating and terrifying.

This state is known medically as 'hyperventilation', and is seen as something to be avoided, which in a sense it obviously is. Yet hyperventilation is the dragon which guards a rich treasure. Physiologically, what is happening is that the person is 'blowing off' carbon dioxide with the outbreath, altering the acid/alkali balance in the bloodstream and thus sending muscles into spasm. This is why an easy and mechanical way to bring someone back to normal is to make them breathe in and out of a paper bag, reabsorbing their own carbon dioxide.

Some medical people draw the conclusion that it is therefore dangerous to breathe deeply! Yet thousands of people have discovered that it is possible to confront and *complete* this process of over-breathing, so that it will not happen again no matter how deeply and strongly we breathe. Over-breathing is a gateway into a world of greater power and sensitivity, and the way through is to dissolve the blocks against expression which set up the tingling and cramps. This is the *energy* level of the process, however we understand it physiologically.

Hands need to grip, to let power move through them, to hit out or to hold on; if they don't they will become cramped, twisted, powerless claws. The voice needs to shout, the mouth to pump the sound out, to say in one way or another 'I'm here, I exist, I feel!' Over-breathing is about *losing control*: either we lose control to paralysis and pain, or we surrender to the free flow of energy and life.

So when over-breathing begins to manifest, we reassure the person that this is a natural healing process, and encourage them to let life flow through the stuck areas. If the stiffness becomes painful, they must yell and groan about that pain! We encourage them to grip on to a blanket with their hands, committing every ounce of their strength, letting power flow down their arms, using their voice to help them grip. As the natural process takes over, sound and movement become natural, spontaneous, releasing. Usually, great waves of pleasure and energy now flow through the previously blocked areas; for a little while, the person floats free on the ocean of being. Such experiences can lead to lasting changes in the bodymind.

At these and other times, some Reichian therapists will use their hands to press on tight muscles in the client. These may be the breathing muscles themselves – the diaphragm, belly and chest – or they may be armoured areas elsewhere in the body which are holding back expression. Pressing, poking, tickling, stretching tight muscles can help them 'overload', so that the charge of feeling spills back into expression. This sort of stimulation usually hurts – and this itself provides a route to expression as the individual reacts to pain with anger, fear or crying. The emotion which comes up will be the one held in the muscle tension.

Pain is a powerful tool in therapeutic bodywork, but it also carries complex implications – about power, for example – and is bound to affect the relationship between client and therapist. Only a few Reichian therapists feel easy about using heavy pressure as a way of *starting* release, though for many clients, as they become more experienced with the work, there are times when they will directly perceive their own holding and welcome the therapist's help in releasing it, even if it does involve pain. The whole area is a complex one, and current realisations about the theme of abuse in life and in therapy make it even more complex – we will look at this issue again in the next chapter. We should perhaps say that the two authors have very different attitudes to strong physical work: Nick sometimes uses it, while Em doesn't.

However, there are many other forms of direct physical interaction which come up in bodywork. As the client follows the sensations and emotions that arise, they often need to push with hands, legs, head, shoulders, pelvis; to hit out at someone (the therapist will hold a cushion in front of herself); to pull against a person's strength; to hold and to be held. In this form of work, the therapist is present with her whole being, body as well as mind, offering herself as a resource, creating an intimacy which, outside sex, is almost unique in adult life.

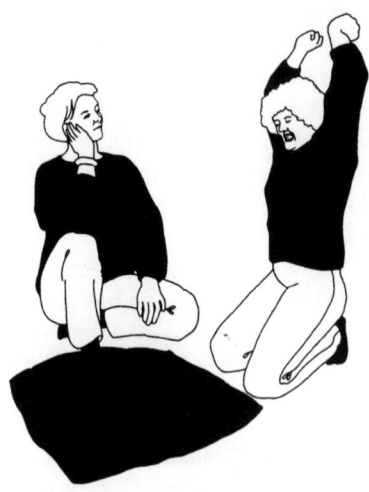

EMOTION

It will be obvious already that the four spheres we are considering overlap with each other. Much of what we have said about the physical body also involves emotions, energy and ideas. Once life force is on the move it functions in all modes at once. We are distinguishing only the different starting points for the process.

On the other hand, emotions and physical sensations have a particularly close link. The word 'feeling' can be used for both kinds of experience, and in practice during a therapy session the client may make no distinction between what they are feeling physically and what they are feeling emotionally. Other people, however, may find it very hard to link the two – it is common to have bodily experiences with no emotional content, or vice versa. You can also find yourself in a separate 'witnessing' part of your being, coolly registering the experience, deducing, 'Ah, now my voice sounds angry/sad/ frightened.' All these are fine as starting points; the goal is to reconnect with the unity of our experience.

Many clients do not feel ready or able to engage with bodywork when they begin therapy. The process seems too intimate, too invasive, perhaps even meaningless to someone who doesn't experience themselves as 'living in' their body.

Thus therapy will always start with the sorts of contact that *are* available, but with the long-term goal of coming to grips with whatever is blocking bodywork. This is not meant to imply that bodywork is more 'fundamental' than other approaches; the same will apply in reverse, for example, with a client who finds bodywork easy but treats it purely physically, making no emotional connections. With a number of clients, then, the starting point will be an exploration of their emotional world, during which the therapist is hoping to bring to their awareness how they resist specific kinds of feeling. Just as bodywork focuses on the muscular armouring against movement and breathing, so here we are looking at character armouring against feeling and expression.

In this sort of work it is crucial that the therapist be in touch with her own feelings and her own defences against feeling, in order to explore those of her client, just as in bodywork we need to be in touch with our own breath. One of our fundamental tools for understanding in this area is registering the emotions which arise within ourselves during the session. These feelings and attitudes will almost always reflect what is going on *inside the client*. To make use of this information, however, we must be clear enough to disentangle it from our own character, our own habits of feeling which will 'rise to the bait'. This is one of many reasons why therapists need to receive regular therapy!

When two people are relating strongly, their emotional states are linked; a feeling in one will produce an echo in the other without anything being explicitly stated. So our internal reactions help us see how the client is resisting feeling, resisting expression. Often a client will insist that 'nothing is happening', no emotions of any sort are being experienced. If the therapist knows herself well, however, she may for example perceive a wave of sadness or of fear which doesn't come from her own process. She can then feed this back to the client: 'I sense a lot of sadness in the room at the moment. Is that to do with what you're telling me about?'

What *doesn't* happen is almost more important than what does. A client may find it very easy to cry, for example, but almost impossible to get angry, or even assertive. The therapist must obviously validate and support the tears, but she must also notice, point out, *insist* on the 'missing feeling' which those tears may be covering up. An apparently inappropriate edge of anger or confrontation within *herself* during the session is an important clue to what is happening. It may also work the other way round: if I feel angry with a client perhaps they are *expecting* me to be angry, almost encouraging it – because this is what they are used to.

Little of the resistance to feeling will be conscious, of course. As we have emphasised, the purpose of armouring is partly to make feelings unconscious. But we still communicate those unacknowledged feelings all the time, and a therapist can be sensitive enough to mirror back the feelings her clients are rejecting in a way which validates their pain and defensiveness, but which also invites and challenges them to re-own their hidden self.

> **Exercise 26**
> You might find it interesting at this point to think about which feelings you yourself find it easy to express – and which ones are unacceptable or unavailable to you. Are you someone who 'never gets angry'? Or are you apparently 'fearless'? Or perhaps you approach most situations in the expectation of being hurt? After you have made your own list, try asking one or two people close to you how they see you – the result may be illuminating.

A slightly different way of seeing the process is that the therapist is throwing the spotlight on whatever behaviour *resists contact*. Character is a system of defence; it rests on the childhood realisation that the world is dangerous, and should not be approached with honest directness. In particular we should not be open with people in authority, which is how the therapist appears. She is dangerous, because she may – indeed, is actively trying to – open up dangerous emotions. Right from the start we, as clients, are unconsciously trying to control the situation, to put limits on it, to make it less spontaneous and contactful, trying in fact to sabotage the therapy which is costing us so much money and effort!

A client may, for example, enter therapy with an apparent deep trust and faith in the therapist's ability to help them: a biddable compliance with all suggestions, and boundless enthusiasm for the results. Wonderful! The unwary therapist basks in the satisfaction of being admired and appreciated, yet somehow nothing seems to lead anywhere; there is no deepening, no discovery. Eventually the therapist is forced to realise that all this trust is inauthentic: the client's real message is 'I'm a good boy/girl, don't hurt me'. When the client can begin to experience their fear and suspicion of the therapist then something real can start to happen.

Another client may begin therapy in a truculent, suspicious and complaining way. Nothing the therapist does is right; no session ends in a satisfying resolved way. It's always left uncertain whether the client will come back next week. Nevertheless they do keep coming back, they must be getting something out of it. Could it be that what they want, yet are fighting, is to surrender, to be small and trusting and looked after?

These are just two examples of the many ways in which people's conscious feelings on entering therapy can be contradicted by deeper motivations. Part of the therapist's job is to look beyond the surface presented to them; not in a distrustful and cynical way, which would simply represent their own character armour, but with heart contact and an awareness of when and how whatever needs to happen isn't happening. Our basic belief is that everyone enters therapy in order to become open – however hard they may resist that openness! As therapists we seek to ally ourselves with that wholesome and authentic aspect of our client, by revealing the wholesome and authentic part of ourselves.

Working to uncover a client's deep feelings involves being in touch with what their bodies are doing, especially their breathing and posture. It means listening to the unconscious messages which may utterly contradict the words they say – 'I feel happy and relaxed', yet my shoulders are tense, my arms folded and my breathing shut down. It also involves looking at their current life situation, often in considerable detail. But even though we expect to spend a good deal of time in the course of our work helping people develop better strategies for managing their lives, therapy is not advice-giving; our main concern with current events is how they illuminate a person's fundamental patterns formed in childhood and earlier, their basic expectations of how the world will be, which function like scripts to direct the course of their lives.

THOUGHT

What we have just been saying about feelings clearly concerns a person's thought processes, their ideas about how things are. Generally, however, we are less concerned with someone's explicit ideas than with their silent *assumptions:* 'You can't expect to get what you want from life', 'Everyone lets me down in the end', 'If I want love I have to earn it', 'Anger only gets you hurt', 'Women are born to suffer', 'A real man never cries'. These are a mere handful of the common assumptions people make about life – any one of which will have fundamental effects upon how they go about things, and therefore upon what happens to them.

Our assumptions tend to be self-fulfilling prophecies. If we believe that everyone is out for themselves, then we will act in a suspicious and self-centred fashion which discourages other people from being open and sharing with us. If we believe that anger will get us hurt, then we can easily create that hurt – by punching a wall instead of a cushion, for example, or simply by the way in which our fear makes us hit out clumsily and awkwardly. If we expect not to get what we want, then we want things we know we can't get. And so on.

> **Exercise 27**
> Try to make a list of your habitual, favourite assumptions about reality, on the lines of the above examples. Do this down one half of a page – quite fast and without thinking about it too much; then opposite each statement, write a contradictory statement. Try saying these out loud, and see what it feels like!

It could be said that this kind of thought is fundamentally a *memory*. Our bodymind remembers the existence-threatening situation which stamped a certain view of life onto us; the tactic which allowed us to survive then becomes our basic strategy for confronting life now. But life changes all the time – we are constantly meeting with new experiences, if we can let ourselves recognise them. Through therapy, we can open up a certain spaciousness in our lives, which involves among other things the capacity to *think* more clearly; to perceive, to reconsider, and often to change, our lifelong assumptions about 'how things are'.

Of course these are not merely intellectual notions: their power comes from their intense *emotional* charge, which is always anchored in the structure of our *bodies*, in the ways that *energy* is allowed to move in us. Yet there is a definite role for the mind in therapy! There are times when it can be crucial to understand the logical flaws in our approach to existence – if for no other reason, to motivate us to carry on with the work despite its discomfort.

This is the constructive aspect of the way in which thinking, operating from our heads, distances us from the immediate authenticity of feeling and sensation. Our capacity for analysis enables us to step back to gain perspective, to witness our own process rather than immersing ourselves in it.

The question is whether this distancing effect is voluntary or involuntary; whether it is simply a flight from the anxiety which feelings and sensations can bring up in us. Many people come to therapy needing to 'get out of their heads' – they have been affected by our culture's emphasis on sterile and exaggerated rationality, and have lost touch with their emotions. As we have stressed, feelings are not open to argument: they are simply *there*, to be lived through and completed.

But other people – or the same people at a different moment in their lives – may be excessively involved in their feelings in an addictive or a flooded way, going round and round the same emotional cycle rather than completing it and moving on. At such a point a therapist might well say 'Yes, that's how you feel, but what do you *think* about that? Do your feelings reflect what is actually happening in the here and now?' The client is thus invited to use their powers of analysis to clarify and peel away fossilised emotional attitudes.

Feelings cannot be *changed* by thoughts. If we try to do this we simply repress them, and throw ourselves into an illusion. But thoughts can help us to understand where feelings come from, help us open up a space between the reality of the feeling and the reality of the situation so that we can start to understand that the feeling refers to things in the past rather than in the present (if this is the case). Knowing this, we are encouraged to work out, express and let go of the old emotion, rather than confusing it with current reality and unconsciously trying to make reality match our feeling.

We must remember too that our head is part of our body, and thoughts are a life function much like digestion or heartbeat. Moving into a 'thought space', with its flavour of cool, distant clarity, is accompanied by a shift in our breathing and posture. The breath tends to become more shallow, and focus in our upper chest rather than our belly. The energy focuses in our upper body and our head; the state of our whole head armouring, and our eyes in particular, will determine to a very large extent how free and clear our thought processes can be – how well we can 'see what's going on'.

We should also mention here the very major role in therapy of fantasy and imagination. Working in any of the ways we describe in this chapter, clients are likely to come up with spontaneous imagery about what they are experiencing – not just visual images, but using any of the sensory channels. To take a few random examples: someone might imagine their body as a tree, with a great snake coiling around the trunk. Or they might suddenly smell smoke, or taste blood in their mouth, or hear the sound of bells. Whatever the imagery that emerges, it will be rooted in that individual's history and life issues: we can see it as a message from the bodymind, couched not in language but in sensation. Working with these fantasies – either within the session, or on your own between sessions – can be a most fruitful way of developing communication with yourself.

ENERGY

In the last section, and throughout this chapter, we have shifted at times into talking about 'energy'. What we can perceive as bodywork, as emotional movement, or a shift of ideas, can also be perceived as a flow of life energy, of orgone. A Reichian therapist may focus on this level, watching the energy shifts in their client as a favourite 'channel' for picking up information about what is going on. We may also work directly to affect the flow of energy, rather than doing this through acting on physical or emotional tension. We may use our hands, for instance, not to press or poke the muscles, but to help energy move into or around the client's body. This is an area where therapy overlaps with what is known as 'hand healing', 'spiritual healing', or 'subtle energy work'.

In fact, as most practitioners of therapeutic touch come to realise, there is no hard and fast line between bodywork and energy rebalancing. Hands that are accustomed to touching bodies become steadily more subtle, hinting and offering rather than insisting; out of this dance another form of interaction will flower, letting us realise that it has been going on all the time. It is impossible for two people, two energy systems, *not* to interact on an energy level.

Apart from focusing and channelling energy through our hands, we can use visualisation and imagery. If we imagine, for instance, a stream of clear blue water flowing through and around us, relaxing and clearing our energy, then this is what will tend to happen; or if we hold in our mind's eye the image of a hot orange sun blazing into our belly, or of a white rose slowly opening in our chests, then the appropriate energy shift is likely to occur.

Many practitioners and healing organisations work with energy while keeping quiet about it — it seems too weird, too unacceptable, to acknowledge openly. Reichian work has always acknowledged the direct role of life energy, and, as we shall see in Chapter 11, Reich even developed a series of devices for concentrating that energy and dissolving the blocks against its natural flow. He was also very much aware that a human being is an 'orgone device' — as is any other living being. Energy streams constantly through our bodyminds, at times pooling and condensing, freezing and stagnating, boiling and flooding. Working with energy is really no different from other levels of therapy; it is just a different emphasis of perception, employing the same fundamental concepts and directions as the other spheres. If the energy within us shifts, then our feeling state, thought processes and body awareness will also shift: the four spheres are all interdependent.

Exercise 28
With coloured pens or crayons, make a picture of your body's energy patterns as you imagine them to be. Try to let yourself loose on this; use lots of different colours. You may want to have a body outline to work with — but remember that your energy also goes outside your skin. This is a nice exercise to do with friends, and to do occasionally over a period of time to see how your pictures change.

THE THERAPY RELATIONSHIP

We have just described the *terrain* of the client–therapist interaction, but this is not the interaction itself. At some stage in the work – perhaps even right at the start – the emphasis shifts crucially from the *content* of the therapy – melting armour, releasing feelings, revising life scripts, channelling energy – to the *form* of the therapy, and the relationship between two people which that form expresses.

A client does a specific piece of therapeutic work, arrives at a new insight, perhaps, a new capacity for handling charge. This is the first level of the work, and essential and valuable in itself. But simultaneously, a second level is operating: the piece of work is also a *transaction* between client and therapist.

Is it, for example, an offering, like an apple for the teacher? Is it asking for praise; or appeasing, trying to buy off criticism? Is there an unconscious goal of shocking the therapist, frightening her off with the horror of the material revealed? Is it a test? Does the client expect to be rejected if she shows her real self? Is she calculatedly – but unconsciously – trying to produce the feelings the therapist expects – or to frustrate those expectations?

How, in other words, does the therapeutic work act as a *container* for the client's love or hate for the therapist, for her fear or anger or seductiveness or need?

All this may seem a bit unlikely, a bit over the top. A therapist in touch with her own core is not going around inviting her clients' love or hate. Yet over and over again, therapists since Freud (and no doubt since the dawn of time) have found these super-intense feelings manifesting in their clients, bending everything to their own ends. They have had the certainty that something *underlies* a superficially straightforward piece of work, something much more difficult and confusing, like a great dark star bending the light from a smaller visible sun. And, even more interestingly, we discover equivalent 'over the top' responses *in ourselves;* we feel an urge to praise or punish, seduce or reject, to need things from and do things to our clients.

This is all most alarming, or would be if we lacked an understanding of what is going on. Freud labelled this process 'transference' because, he said, the client is essentially *transferring* on to the therapist powerful positive or negative feelings which were originally called forth by the important adults in their childhood. The equivalent feelings in the therapist are generally known as 'counter-transference'.

The fundamental emotions about people which we had in childhood are the ones we tend to have about all the important people in our lives, not just our therapists. If we were afraid of our parents' anger, we will be afraid of our lovers' anger – whether they get angry or not. And so on with all our other feelings and relationships: rather than being able to see other people directly, we tend to treat them as a screen on to which we project old memories, or current feelings of our own which we would rather not recognise. In the therapy situation, however, there are important and creative differences.

The therapist is not, like most people, simply putting her own projections back onto the client. In the rest of her life, she may project as readily as the next person, but she has learnt not to do so in the therapy session; or rather, to keep a distance from her projections, and to use them as information about what is happening within the client.

Also, in therapy both people are there not for any practical or emotional purpose, which would take their attention away from the projecting that is going on (and often sabotaging that main purpose). They are there simply in order to experience and consider what happens between them. There is plenty of space for projections to arise, develop, play themselves through. There is space for the 'transference relationship' to reveal itself, and thus to reveal the fundamental patterns and assumptions of our lives.

In classic Freudian psychoanalysis, the basic situation that arouses a lot of transference feelings is one of *absence*. The therapist distances herself from the client in all sorts of ways: by sitting out of sight and much of the time in silence, by withholding information about herself and her feelings, by offering little expression of sympathy or concern. The psychoanalyst, at least in theory, is a 'blank screen' on to which the clients project their central feelings about people – especially about people who withhold themselves!

The basis of our own work is crucially different. Although there are some important boundaries in our relationship with clients (for instance, we are offering only a specified amount of time), we are always moving towards *contact*. It is this active push for closeness, for deep disclosure, which provokes transference feelings – as a defence against the power and vulnerability of this contact.

Because it is the relationship with the therapist which provokes such deep feelings, as clients we find it easier to see *them* as responsible for *our* process; to see them as powerful, rather than recognising that the power resides equally in us and in the contact we are both experiencing; to see them as special – specially nice or specially nasty – rather than facing them as simply another human being like us. Contact is only truly possible between equals.

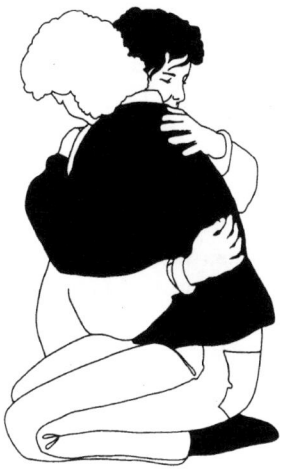

Transference feelings develop in the course of therapy as a last ditch defence against real, equal human contact. This is why it is such a positive and creative movement. The client's unconscious resistance, their character armour, is throwing everything into the battle, manifesting all its skills of defence, evasion and control. Anything is better than the aching vulnerability of spontaneous openness! If the therapist can unwaveringly hold out this option of openness, then the client is forced to see through their illusions about who the therapist is, forced face to face with the deep childhood hurt that has crippled their capacity to be intimate and powerful.

In this intense process the therapist is no unmoved onlooker, no 'objective' technician. She, too, will be stirred to the core; all her residual unwillingness to be open, equal and spontaneous will come to the surface, all her buttons will be pressed as the client with great unconscious skill and insight, tries to throw her off balance, to turn her from a healthy, contactful being into a manifestation of the client's childhood damage and adult expectations.

The counter-transference is the experience of being a puppet for the client's fears and expectations – usually both at once. What lays us open to this is our own unresolved childhood material; especially, of course, the distorted feelings that have contributed to our desire to be therapists in the first place – the need to help people, to have power, to be appreciated.

If we can stay in touch with our wholesome, rational core, we can see the counter-transference impulses for what they are. They then become a treasury of information about the client, as we realise that our tendency to fall in love with them, or bully them, or pass judgement on them, or feel inadequate with them, is something that *they* are doing: a familiar pattern which they are trying to impose on the situation, mainly because it feels safer than the unknown territory of openness.

So what we do with this information is, in one way or another, to feed it back to the client. The therapist's ultimate resource is her capacity to be *honest* – with herself, with her clients, about what is actually going on. This is really the only way to avoid becoming what the client fears yet tries to create – an oppressive authority figure, withholding knowledge as a source of power.

The therapist does not always need to be in control. We have both had so many experiences of losing our balance in a session, getting hot and bothered, being on the edge of panic, and have learnt that we can resolve the whole situation and return effortlessly to centre with some simple statement like 'I feel confused, I don't know what's going on here'. The client's transference reaction tries to make us into someone who *always* knows what's going on, for good or ill – a parent – someone unreal. Being honest and being real is a minimum condition for being therapeutic. In doing this, we are also modelling for our client the possibility of being fluid in one's approach to life, of moving between positions rather than attempting to freeze and rigidify.

It should be clear by now that clients' patterns of transference will match their favoured character positions. Character is a defence against spontaneity and contact; it is the force in us which produces transference as a last ditch defence. So, for example, someone in the Boundary position will experience the therapist's offer of contact as a threat to their existence; will perhaps 'go away inside', be unable to hear or understand properly what is being said to them. In the Oral position, we will feel ourselves as needing to be looked after by the therapist – see them as provider or withholder of nourishment, a 'good' or 'bad' mother. Holding characters will expect to be rejected if they let their feelings show. Thrusting characters will compete for power. Crisis characters will try to stir the therapist up, to unseat or panic them, as a way of unloading their own intolerable panic about contact.

There is a special relationship between the crisis character and transference, since this position is *about* contact, manifesting a yes/no anxiety around the issue. When someone is strongly in this position at the start of therapy, their relationship with the therapist will immediately take on a central role – sometimes before even entering the room for the first time.

In a sense we could say that we all have to pass through this position as part of our therapeutic process. Therapy will stir up our tendencies to each character position in turn, but it is at the 'crisis stage' that the transference relationship becomes crucially important. Can we move through to an open way of relating to our therapist? Can we allow our feelings and sensations, our thoughts and energy, to arise without making the therapist responsible for them? Can we allow the therapist to have *their* feelings without us having to take them on? If so, we have an excellent model for living a sane and creative life outside therapy – which, of course, is the point of the whole exercise.

GOALS

That last sentence may beg a few questions. What *are* the goals of therapy? Clients may come to a therapist for all sorts of reasons, conscious and unconscious. What is therapy *for?* Where are we trying to get to through these practices and procedures?

The longer we work as therapists, the more we find our original goals fading away, revealing themselves as illusions. The first to go was an intention of 'helping people', 'making it better'. This soon revealed itself as not only impossible to achieve, but actually harmful to attempt. If I try to 'help' you, I am defining you as helpless, myself as helpful – a systematic disempowerment which undermines your attempts at freedom and independence, plays straight into the transference defence, and encourages me in my delusions of grandeur!

Nor is therapy really even about people getting *better* – if by 'better' we mean their physical or emotional ills dissolving, their life becoming happier and more successful. These things do very often happen – clients gain in acceptance, confidence, creativity, capacity for pleasure in sex and life in general; serious physical ailments clear up; chronic pains disappear. These, of course, are the sorts of things people hope for when they start therapy.

However, we have to face the fact that all these things are essentially by-products of therapy rather than the thing itself. Occasionally a person will end therapy feeling that it has been valuable and successful, and their therapist will agree, yet the original problem, their reason for coming, may be quite untouched. It is not uncommon that during therapy a person's relationship may break up; a life situation which previously felt fine becomes intolerable; they can even manifest new and major physical ailments. Yet they may well still feel positive about the therapeutic process. Is this a tribute to our powers of brainwashing? We don't believe so.

Therapy helps people to face reality; it helps them discover what reality *is*, to let go of illusions. At the end of this process – or rather, at the end of this phase of a never-ending process – life may feel easier or harder, tragic or ecstatic. But the person will be more in touch with their own process, their own self. They will be in contact with 'what they came for', and working out the implications as fully as possible. Occasionally, as Arnold Mindell says, the successful resolution of a therapeutic process is for the client to *die*.

We don't have a lot of clients dying at the end of therapy, though it is true that a very extreme level of defence can manifest as a person's core starts to surface. The point we are trying to make is that although therapy allows a person's life to deepen, to become *richer*, it does not necessarily make it *easier*. They may have spent their lives ignoring and avoiding pain, both inside and out in the real world. That pain is real; heartbreak is real; exhaustion and death are real. In an initial interview with a prospective client, it may often seem that the therapist is trying to put the client off rather than encouraging them.

It may be better to speak of *directions* for therapy rather than goals – at any moment in the process of working with someone, our direction will be towards more honesty, more spontaneity, more openness, more energy, more space. Whether the specific experiences this brings out are 'good' or 'bad' is irrelevant, as long as our belief and our experience is that the core of a human being is loving, joyful and creative. As therapists, our work is to midwife the birth of this core.

Can therapy fail? Certainly it can. At times there seem to be so many layers of negative emotion around the clear core that we despair of ever reaching it, and this can be as true of ourselves as of other people. The world we live in is not exactly a welcoming home, or even a *possible* home, for open individuals. People give up and leave; the therapist can give up and send them away, directly or indirectly. Yet even then who can say that the process is over? It often goes on working inside someone; they may come back to therapy with the same practitioner or someone else, or find some other tool, or simply live their lives in a different and more complete way. The idea of 'reaching the core' is really an illusion anyway: we are already there. If therapy is, or tries to be, a natural process, then like the rest of nature it is never complete, never wholly separate – never, really, 'good' or 'bad'.

BEING A THERAPIST; BEING A CLIENT

What we have said may make it seem that a therapist is a saint-like being, one who has resolved all her own childhood feelings and become a permanently open character. Luckily this is not the case, or there would be a striking shortage of therapists!

What the activity *does* require is a practised ability to put one's own material on one side for the duration of the session, except in so far as it becomes an important part of what is going on. People often talk about the therapist 'leaving her own problems outside the door'; in our experience it is much more a question of constantly owning up to and releasing the feelings which arise in us. Most of the time we can do this silently and quickly, but when we hit a bigger issue it is vital that we don't try to conceal it or unload it onto the client. We must be able to own up to what is going on – and this is not so much a precondition for therapy; it *is* the therapy.

Thus giving therapy to someone else is a bit like giving it to yourself. It becomes a form of meditation, repeatedly coming back to clear attention in the here and now, to focusing on the other person's experience without ever giving up or denying your own humanity. The most important thing is that being a therapist is just an activity, like any other activity which is useful and satisfying.

What *do* we get out of giving therapy? Most therapists are rather nosey people, who like to know what's going on for everyone. Many of us have a tendency, usually reasonably well-controlled, to enjoy feeling important, bossing people around, 'helping'. Giving therapy can also be a very effective defence against our own therapeutic process – shifting attention away from ourselves and on to other people. A lot of therapists tend to reach a plateau in their work on themselves and stay there.

It is crucial that therapists continue to get regular therapy for themselves, or find other ways of continuing to explore and grow, so as to remain clear about their own motivations and their own process. We have noticed a distinct relationship between our work on ourselves and our work with other people: if one becomes frustrating, so does the other, and if one becomes creative, so does the other. Every therapist is also a client.

And being a client can also become a career! You can become addicted to therapy: use it in many subtle ways as a means of shoring up your defended character rather than challenging it. Every therapist meets the 'professional client' who has done a bit of everything, and now wants to add you to their trophies.

With therapy, as with every other human activity that tends towards liberation, there is a constant gravitational pull back into unreality, back into routine. The fact that we have to do it for money as a profession is one factor here – 'Oh God, back to work'. For clients and therapists alike there is the constant challenge to renew the process, to come back to the core, back to simplicity, back to naturalness, back to freedom.

GROUPS

In this chapter we have been talking essentially about therapy in the 'classic' setting – a one-to-one relationship, usually for an hour a week, and lasting for some months or years. There are many other possible settings. Reich himself worked like most psychoanalysts, seeing clients for an hour three to five times a week. Very few people could afford such an arrangement in the milieux in which we work.

Partly because of cost, partly because of other power issues which we shall look at in the next chapter, and partly because of other advantages, we do a great deal of work in groups: day, weekend or longer workshops, usually centred around people *exchanging* Reichian sessions in pairs, with the support and supervision of one or two leaders moving between the pairs.

The great strengths of this kind of work (developed by William West, largely under the influence of the Co-Counselling movement, and also of Peter Jones) are that it is cost- and labour-effective, and it is *empowering*, proving to people that they have the capacity to care, to give, to share. Giving such a session can itself be an important therapeutic experience. Also, the sheer amount of energy generated in a room full of Reichian sessions tends to intensify the work and increase the likelihood of stirring and worthwhile things happening.

At the same time, it is obvious that this structure limits the sort of work which is possible. Generally speaking the emphasis will be on bodywork, because in this sphere the client is more 'self-starting' through focusing on the breath. The bodywork is inevitably reduced to a few clear, simple principles, since many of the helpers may never have worked therapeutically before; indeed they may never before have touched another person's body in a non-sexual way.

It might seem as though the structure of pair work would have less value than working with a therapist or might even be dangerous. This is by no means the case. The emphasis becomes one of 'being there': the helper's main role is to give supportive attention, to let the person working know that someone is with them and that whatever they are experiencing is all right. Any further assistance depends on the skills and confidence of the helpers, some of whom may have attended several groups and be quite experienced and sensitive. The group leaders are there to handle tricky moments and deal with stuckness.

Running groups is in many ways a humbling experience for a practising therapist. It puts our skills and theories back in proportion, showing us just how much can be done through the willingness to be open and to give attention. The distinction between 'therapist' and 'ordinary person' is a purely practical one – by earning our living at this work we develop a great deal of experience, but also lose out somewhat in freshness and commitment. Running a group can be a bit like giving an exhibition of simultaneous chess! But at other times there may be nothing for the leader to do at all.

Especially during a longer group, the more verbal, 'character-analytic' side of the work will develop, through time spent with the whole group together, sitting in a circle, with people taking turns to share and explore what is going on for them with the help of the leaders and of other members of the group. The group itself becomes a resource for its members, a source of healing and growth, with its own inherent wisdom and sense of direction.

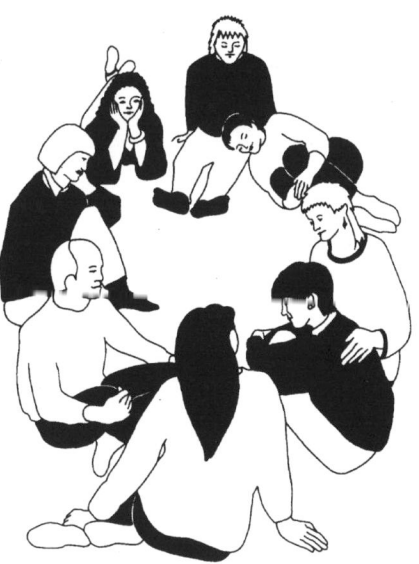

A group is also capable of very powerful negative and destructive feelings. On rare occasions, especially during long-term groups, a 'mob' atmosphere can develop, as hostile transference feelings towards the leaders, or the scapegoating of certain group members, becomes amplified by positive feedback. This is the sort of situation where a therapist needs all her capacity for centredness and constructive honesty, yet the possibility of deep core contact is correspondingly amplified by the group situation, and many very beautiful and magical experiences can occur.

9

Power

> Love, work and knowledge are the wellsprings of our life; they should also govern it.
>
> Wilhelm Reich

Reading what we have said about the client–therapist relationship, many people will be concerned about issues of power. Is it acceptable for therapists to work in a way which deliberately lets them become such charged figures for their clients? Isn't there a tremendous potential in this situation for exploitation? Isn't the relationship structured so as inevitably to disempower the client, stripping away their autonomy and identity rather than strengthening them?

These are serious questions, and ones which make quite a few people steer clear of therapy, Reichian or otherwise, however much they may in some ways be drawn to it. The ultimate fear is similar to that felt about the Moonies or the Rajneesh movement – of a Svengali-like, mesmeric figure who controls our actions and perceptions.

This is a highly rational fear in a society where a great deal of time and money is devoted to controlling people's actions and perceptions. Just as our culture is manipulative in the public sphere, through advertising and propaganda, so in the private sphere people assert coercive power over each other's experience. This is especially brutal between parents and children where the child's reality can be forcibly invalidated and invaded, both physically and mentally. We don't even have to look at the sickening facts of extreme abuse; incest and torture are the logical extension of the powerless situation in which most children find themselves in our culture.

The intense vulnerability which therapy exposes will often bring up these sorts of childhood feelings and memories. It is all too easy for the therapist to push away her own distress by pushing around the client, instructing her in subtle or not-so-subtle ways what to think and feel and remember. Therapists can easily become addicted to the power thrust upon them by so many clients, who have themselves been brought up to 'need' an authority to obey: therapists can actually start *believing* in the positive transference they receive. Acting in this way is equally abusive, however nice it feels.

There are some therapists, and some therapies, which tend to exploit their clients, emotionally, financially, or by imposing a social 'norm' upon the client's experience. Suspicions of exploitation, like any other conflicts of perception between the two people involved, need to be carefully and thoroughly examined, *without* any built-in assumption that the therapist is more likely to be 'right' than the client.

It is the therapist's willingness to test out her own attitudes and feelings, and on occasion to own up to mistakes and confusions, which can above all make therapy a safe and non-abusive structure. As we have tried to show in the last chapter, by working as therapists we are not setting ourselves up as superior beings. People often describe the therapy relationship as 'unequal'. We don't think this is right, we see it more as 'asymmetrical' – the roles of the two people are not the same, and their involvement is of different kinds. But the *power* of the participants can and must balance.

This goal is on its own a radical and subversive one in a society which is constructed out of inequalities of power. Our work is very much concerned with the difference between 'power-over' and 'power-for'; with helping the client to feel this difference in her own marrow. Power-over is the juice upon which patriarchal culture runs – the assumption that if I am strong, someone else must be weak, and vice versa. This is part of the myth of scarcity, which says that there isn't enough of anything, so we must all fight for our share of the inadequate cake.

Scarcity is only a truth about the things our culture has created to be scarce: luxuries, or money itself. It isn't even a truth that *food* is scarce, only that it is unevenly distributed; and it isn't remotely true of breath, energy, love or power – in the sense of power-for-ourselves, strength and creativity, 'the force that through the green fuse drives the flower' as Dylan Thomas puts it.

There is plenty of power for everyone!

But patriarchal society cannot allow this reality to be felt, otherwise no one would let their power apparently be taken away, no one would bow down to their 'betters', or work in a boring and useless job, or obey silly rules, or let other people control all the resources and activities of society, or let our shared environment be degraded and damaged. Social oppression depends ultimately on *consent*: we let it happen.

Why do we consent to being disempowered in this way? Reich was one of the first people to point out the vital role of family life in transmitting patriarchal ideas and ways of being. We are made controllable by our *armouring*, which walls off so much of our energy, clarity, courage and initiative. While many people would see this as 'healthy discipline', we see it as an *education in disempowerment*. And this same armouring, by blocking our urge for loving contact so that it turns stagnant and vicious, sets up the conditions for people to be attracted by the violence, hatred and scapegoating of fascism and other extreme ideologies.

Authority: public and private

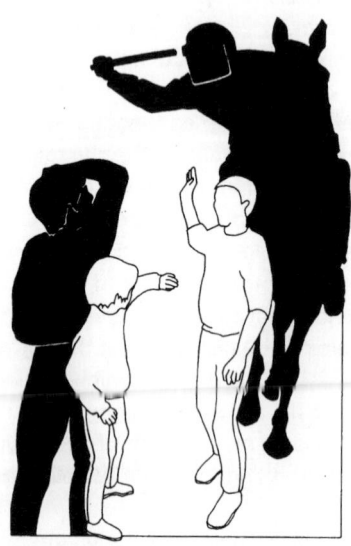

We can draw real parallels between different political ideologies and the different layers of the armoured personality. The liberal/democratic consensus, denying the reality of oppression and exploitation, corresponds to the outer layer of false 'niceness' and 'civilisation'. Extremist ideologies of the right and left, with all their talk of 'smashing', 'liquidating', 'seizing' and 'fighting', correspond to the Middle Layer – the welter of hateful and distorted feelings created through the frustration of our need for love and pleasure. Like all symptoms they have a double nature, expressing both the sadistic rage of a suppressed individual and the compulsive obedience instilled by the authoritarian parenting which suppresses them.

And the healthy core? It corresponds to a way of life which exists so far only in our dreams, one which is not 'political' in the usual sense, because all power remains with the individual and the community, where people control their own lives and work, without needing neurotically to give that control away to 'specialists'. This is the social version of natural self-regulation within the individual.

Of course, it is perfectly possible to 'struggle' and 'fight' for this sort of society by means which are neurotic and distorted! Over and over again, in the public sphere, wonderful visions of freedom and healing have resulted in totalitarian or chaotic societies. It seems pretty clear that it is not possible for armoured characters like ourselves to create a healthy society: either we end up giving our power away to another bunch of brutal authorities, or else we are unable to focus enough creative energy to get anything done at all!

So is there any alternative to doomed attempts at pulling ourselves up by our own bootstraps? Reichian therapy seeks to intervene at the other end of the process of political oppression: to expose the precise distortions created in our individual energies, and to dissolve them so that energy can move freely again.

Reichian therapy makes people less easy to control! They become at least partially immune to manipulation through guilt, shame, anxiety and greed, because these secondary emotions have dissolved back into their primary sources: love, anger, grief, fear and joy. Energy is on the move, and will no longer fit into constricting and damaging containers: bad relationships, bad jobs, bad belief systems. Without any ideology being imposed from outside, the natural forces of the human organism create change in the political situation of the individual: a process of re-empowerment.

However creative, this falling away of a familiar context can be very painful for an individual. Established support systems and friendships often become unsatisfying, no longer able to meet the need for new and different sorts of emotional feeding. Increasingly, we are seeing the need for support networks, ways in which people can validate and aid this sort of change in each other.

But it would take a very long time to change the world through individual or group therapy. We must clearly recognise that therapy becomes a real need, or even a real option, *only* when basic needs for food, housing, security and so on have been met. In this sense, therapy does tend to be a middle-class, privileged activity (though by no means all our clients fall into this group). Thus it is a good thing that, however messianic we become at times, this work is only one tributary of a much greater streaming of change and rebirth. What we see happening over and again is that people move from therapy with us into *other* areas of transformative activity; above all, they begin to change their own lives into an environment where they, and everyone around them, can flower.

Therapy also has a valuable input to make into other forms of working for change. It helps people to examine their *motives* in taking on such tasks; helps them let go of the compulsiveness about 'helping', the workaholism, the hidden authoritarianism or the oral demandingness ('give us our rights!') which can blight so much radical work. Therapy insists that we can and must *enjoy* ourselves; that pleasure and fun are just as much part of changing the world.

It can also suggest new structures and procedures for meetings, co-operatives and so on, based on recognising and giving space to each person involved; paying attention to atmospheres and unspoken agendas rather than sweeping them under the carpet; creating opportunities for personal, face-to-face contact; giving control of work to the people who actually carry it out. Such structures both grow out of and help to nurture natural self-regulation and being-in-touch.

Reichian therapy has a particular natural affinity for two issues of power: sexism and ecology. Reich was, again, one of the first people to raise issues that now come under the banner of 'ecology'. He perceived the spreading pollution and damage to nature in the early 1950s and linked it directly with the blocking of natural impulses in human beings – only armoured and distressed individuals would permit their environment to be poisoned. Therapy tends to liberate feelings of identification with the other-than-human world, the sense of sacredness which most of us lose touch with in childhood, and which makes it impossible to tolerate the rape and torture of the earth.

That image of rape brings us to the issue of sexism: the oppression of natural and spontaneous feeling under patriarchy is tied up in many ways with gender and sex. As we have already said, the wholeness of our experience is split in two by the imposition of 'masculine' and 'feminine' categories of behaviour, creating a permanent wound in both genders, but particularly a structural oppression and devaluation of the female gender. It is no coincidence that nature itself is associated with the female: most of us have deep-ingrained connections between 'female', 'natural', 'animal', 'dirty', 'sexual' and 'wrong'. These ideas are not remotely natural themselves, but are the product of a society which glorifies an equally unnatural constellation of 'male', 'technological', 'human', 'clean', 'intellectual' and 'right'.

Sexism is always a powerful presence in therapy because, perhaps more than any other form of social control and oppression, it affects our *bodily* experience. As we have already hinted, many forms of 'symptom' or 'illness' can be understood as a *rebellion* against imposed realities – against abuse of one sort or another. As therapists we want to side not with the parental role, either the 'good' or the 'bad' parent, but with the confused and damaged child itself, and with its never-ending struggle for loving contact. This can often mean retranslating the 'problem' with which the client arrives into the beginning of a 'solution'. This is especially true when the 'problem' is about someone's inability to conform to sexist criteria of normality.

The therapy session is a very unusual sort of space, very different in many ways from 'ordinary life'. One big difference is that the focus of both people's attention is on the experience of one of them – the client. In one sense this makes the client powerful, central. In another sense, it means that the therapist is not exposing her own pain and vulnerability, so she can *appear* always clear and strong. We regularly draw attention to this as we are giving therapy, and make it apparent – without using the client's time for our own needs – that we too feel weak, confused, armoured, stuck in childhood patterns, and so on.

During the session, we are not *being* these things. We have made a contract to focus on the client, knowing that we are able in most situations to keep a clear perspective on our own material when it surfaces. But we couldn't do this if we weren't getting support ourselves at other times, opportunities to panic, fall apart, act irrationally, be totally selfish. We have our own moments, many moments, of vulnerability and lack of clarity in our lives.

We don't try to fool any client about this; in a sense we want to draw their attention to it as part of the human context of our interaction. We will, however, avoid any tendency to turn the spotlight on ourselves during the session, just as with any other avoidance of the client's own feelings and experiences, except when it becomes necessary for both people to spend time sorting out the origins of our own responses to the client.

What happens in therapy, although different, cannot be separated off from the rest of life; which is basically a good thing, since otherwise it could hardly affect the rest of life. One aspect of this is that we are almost invariably taking money from clients for the work we do. This is necessary in order for us to live, and it also creates innumerable opportunities for bad power relationships.

For some clients, the financial relationship increases their sense of the therapist's powerfulness. Not only are we seeing into their souls, we're also taking their cash! There is a sense, though, in which by paying us the client is asserting her control, her choice, in the situation – she is acting as our 'employer'. This too, of course, can be turned into a messy game if the client tries to control our behaviour, perhaps using money as a weapon.

In some ways it might be simpler and cleaner if money did not have to change hands. We don't really subscribe to the convenient notion that 'clients wouldn't value the work if they didn't have to pay for it'. At the same time, though, we live in a world where money is a vital element of exchange and survival, and therapy is to do with recognising reality. Also, there are certainly advantages in having a therapeutic relationship in which the state has no role of subsidy – and therefore of control. We have not resolved the tension between our need for a reasonable standard of living and our desire to work with people irrespective of their level of income. Group therapy provides a very partial solution, and we certainly see it as necessary to at least try to offer some cheap sessions.

The issue of money is just one of the many ways in which our practice of Reichian therapy is constantly struggling with contradictions around issues of power. Although we are looking for contact with our clients, and not aiming to withhold ourselves, we still set up very definite boundaries – of time, of disclosure – and some people find these very unsatisfactory. Although we see our work as having a 'public', political dimension, we are still working in 'private' and professional structures, still involved much of the time with the need to generate income, to attract punters!

These contradictions are not going to disappear. Like so many other problems in life, we are going to have to live with them. It feels important to admit that they are there, yet in each situation still to work concretely to move away from 'power-over' and towards 'power-for'.

10

Primal Patterns

> ... What we're pressing after now was once nearer and truer and attached to us with infinite tenderness. Here all is distance, there it was breath. Compared with that first home the second seems ambiguous and draughty.
>
> Rainer Maria Rilke, *Duino Elegies*

In some ways this chapter belongs straight after those on 'character', but we have left it until now to give you a rest from trying to absorb ways of looking at people! It's helpful as well to have some idea of what goes on in therapy in order to grasp these strange experiences which emerge from it. The ideas in this chapter are not part of 'mainstream' Reichian work, but very much a later development; however, they grow largely out of things that happen to people during Reichian sessions.

At the end of Chapter 6, we talked a little about 'regression' and 'progression', which are bound up with the fact that, at every point in life, we are internally busy reinterpreting *the present in terms of the past and the past in terms of the present*.

This is such an important concept that we want to pause for a moment for you to absorb it. We reinterpret the present in terms of the past, and the past in terms of the present.

We reinterpret the present in terms of the past. This is one of the central points that therapy makes: past experience of pain and vulnerability will dispose us to react defensively to new experiences – to assume that they are 'just the same' as what happened in the past. The burnt child dreads the fire. The system of character analysis is a way of finding patterns in this process, which happens not just in our minds but equally in our bodies. Not all of the past is painful, of course – experiences of joy, nurturing and safety will dispose us to approach the present openly and bravely.

We reinterpret the past in terms of the present. This is a more difficult but perhaps equally important idea. New experiences can and do break through into our awareness and reactivate, 'wake up', experiences from the past which seem to have a similar structure; difficult experiences which until now we have managed to tolerate, or positive experiences which we have discounted. We are constantly, unconsciously, re-writing our stories, re-reckoning our lives. This goes on all through adulthood, but especially in the early years when our characteristic approach to existence, the underlying bodymind beliefs, are still being formed.

If we can hold these two ideas firmly in mind, then it helps us to see why it is that very much the *same* character types we have described are seen by many therapists and psychoanalysts as being established in the first weeks or months of life, rather than in the first six or seven years as we have argued. In fact, some people derive all these character positions from what happens during birth itself – or even in the womb before birth.

One can make out a vivid, plausible case for each of these viewpoints, just as we feel we have made out a good case for the crucial role of developmental phases up to about five. If we focus on birth, or on early breastfeeding relationships, or on the details of conception, implantation and gestation, we see the same patterns, the same choices, clearly delineated.

How extraordinary! Or is it? Right along our lifeline we are the same human organism, living in the same universe, and one of our basic human capacities is to make patterns and to hold those patterns through and across time.

Freud very rightly says that in the unconscious there is *no time*; no past, no future. It is an illusion to imagine that because one event is 'earlier' on an individual's lifeline, it therefore causes events which happen 'later'. Our internal pattern-maker is constantly adjusting, re-evaluating, totalising, synthesising, condensing, so as to create a new whole.

Someone who is crushed by adult authority over the issue of toilet training, say, will pattern this experience together with that of being squeezed intolerably in the birth canal. Someone who swallows their anger at age four because they are afraid to rage at their parents will synthesise this guilt with their feelings of hating – yet also helplessly loving – their mother's breast at six months, with a sense of being poisoned in the womb by toxins from their mother's bloodstream, or a sense of being 'fed rubbish' by a dogmatic therapist whom, nonetheless, they dare not alienate by criticism.

As human beings, we use all our experiences as metaphors or examples of each other, creating what the therapist Stanislav Grof calls 'COEX Systems' (systems of COndensed EXperience). We can imagine great balls of clustered memories and feelings, brought together around the magnetism of a shared theme, a primal 'colour'

– loss, for example, or helplessness, or expansion, or security. These COEX systems exist not just in our minds, but also in our bodies, in the patterns of bodily expectation and defence which constitute our armouring.

We can make these difficult ideas more concrete by taking up an example that arises regularly in our work, the experience of *birth.*

Many therapists and growth workers have discovered that it is fairly easy to facilitate a bodymind experience in most people which to everyone involved will seem like a 'birth'. We use quotation marks because we don't believe that people are necessarily re-experiencing a birth that they actually *had*. We think more in terms of what we call a 'birth-shaped experience'; and it really *is* birth-shaped, as many mothers, midwives and obstetricians can testify who have witnessed and experienced it.

There are many effective ways to set up a birthing experience, some much more elaborate than others. What we ourselves generally do is to lay someone on a mattress, curled up on their side, with a blanket over them. One helper puts both hands on the crown of the birthee's head and gives a gentle rhythmic pressure, another helper does the same with the feet, while one or two more people lie on or against the birthee's body to give a sense of enclosure and pressure.

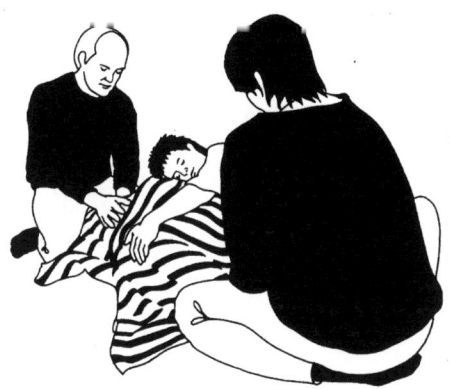

Then we wait – for as long as it takes. It is crucial that the birthing should be initiated and shaped by the birthee; only then will it feel like an authentic event. Sometimes there will be a long wait; nothing apparently happens, at least from the outside viewpoint. There are a few small movements under the blanket, once or twice the breathing will deepen and strengthen, only to fade away again.

Inside the 'womb', however, a great deal may be going on. The birthee moves in and out of an altered state of consciousness; many strange and confusing feelings, images and memories flow through them. Eventually, there develops a genuine urge to *push*, which has a truly involuntary and spontaneous quality, and is often preceded by a build-up of powerful circular breathing (breathing with no pause between inhale and exhale).

Once the birthee begins to push, it is for the helpers to follow and match the impetus which they experience from the birthee; to judge with their bodies more than with their minds the amount of pressure and resistance which is needed, how 'hard' or 'easy' the birth needs to be, whether a 'midwife' needs to go in and pull the birthee out. The experience becomes extraordinarily real and vivid for those taking part and when the 'baby' is finally 'born' between the legs of the helper who has been holding their head, and lies floppy and dazed on someone's lap, perhaps sucking at their hand, it is a moving, heart-opening experience, and it can be hard to keep in mind that this newborn creature is in fact an adult woman or man.

Birthing creates a magic space, an altered state for everyone involved. Only afterwards do people wake up and realise how far they have travelled from everyday reality. Such experiences carry their own conviction, and often have profound effects on the lives of those who pass through them, as they gain a new level of energy and joy in their lives, a more vivid sense of reality, a sense of being truly reborn.

They will also often have learnt specific lessons from the birthing about their basic life patterns. They may now understand in a new way their tendency to push blindly through difficulties, or their constant urge to give up, or the feeling that 'no one's there for me', or the sense that something always goes wrong at the last minute.

All these traits and many others can be illuminated by seeing them as generalisations which we have built up from our experience of being born. There are indeed times, as we have experienced when we have been dealing with a series of birthings in the course of our work, when *everything* about life seems to reflect our birth! We become acutely sensitive to phrases like 'a tight spot', 'cutting our ties', 'no way out', 'light at the end of the tunnel'.

There are often quite specific details of the birthing which relate to obstetrical events: the cord round the neck, the breech presentation, the high forceps, the delayed breathing, the caesarean section – all these emergencies can be reproduced in a birthing. Sometimes they match well with the biographical facts – even when the birthee only consciously discovers the details later.

At other times, though, the events of the birthing will be quite different from what actually happened, and when we go through a second, or third, or subsequent birthing, it is often the case that the whole shape of the experience will be quite different from the first time. It seems that each of us is 'programmed' with a whole series of births, from the most beautiful and joyful to the most horrifically life-threatening, and with a need to experience and release all these births at different times.

So what is going on here? No one really knows, but it appears that the crucial experience of being born – perhaps the first great crisis of life (though there are those who emphasise conception and implantation) – remains as a kind of *resource* for the child and adult, a vocabulary of fundamental feeling-shapes through which we express the later events of life. Each subsequent crisis will summon up for our internal pattern-maker a particular aspect of birth: magnify it, altering the biographical reality, even develop a largely imaginary birth which will then function in our bodymind as if it had really happened.

This is speculation, but what we do know is that the 'birth-shaped experience' quite often happens *spontaneously* in therapy, with no need for any setting up on the therapist's part. We have learnt in practice to spot the signs that a client is moving into such an experience: a need to push with their head and neck, statements like 'I feel there's something I have to get through' or 'something big is going on but I don't understand it': most of all a specific atmosphere, which is hard to describe but highly recognisable – a dreamlike, sleepy premonition which seems to fill the room. In such situations we simply offer our experience and our bodies as resources for the client to shape their own birthing, and save the analysis for afterwards.

And, of course, these birth-shaped experiences happen in *life*. Most human cultures apart from ours have a formal place for 'rites of passage' to mark crucial transitions – puberty, marriage, death, initiation – and these are modelled on birth. The central figure goes down into a dark enclosed place and comes back up into life; is immersed in water; undergoes an ordeal. Even without this ritual enactment we all experience crisis and transition as a death and rebirth, passing through a strait and narrow place.

Another set of images which come up both in and out of therapy are clustered around the umbilical cord and its cutting: ideas of being *connected* to someone or something – fed by them or helplessly poisoned with bad stuff, ideas of being cut off, abandoned, irretrievably damaged. 'Cord-shaped experiences' recur in a variety of situations, and seem to set off reactions which are outside our conscious control.

Again, such themes are anchored in our *bodies*. Massaging around the navel can bring up very powerful feelings, especially of rage and grief, and also fear of falling – our basic sense of grounding seems to be anchored in the umbilical connection, only later being transferred to the legs and the earth. After someone has been birthed and is lying peacefully in a helper's arms, there is sometimes a moment of sudden shock, pain and disorientation which seems to represent the cutting of the cord – often done brutally soon, before it has naturally stopped pulsing as the breath takes over. Almost everyone who goes through the birthing experience emerges as a supporter of natural childbirth and an opponent of high-tech obstetrics.

Another very striking feature of the birth-shaped experience is that, time and again, it spontaneously throws up 'past life memories'. Once more, the quotation marks are to indicate that we are not assuming these indicate a 'real' previous incarnation, simply that after birthing many people emerge with clear and strong images of being someone else in another time and place. These images may parallel the birthing experience itself – for example, someone may envision a death by strangling during a birthing where breathing is difficult.

This sort of experience can be very startling – even annoying, to a person who is sceptical about reincarnation! But like birthing itself, past life imagery can be useful in helping people to make sense of and resolve present issues, helping them create a coherent 'story of themselves'. It is also possible to become addicted to past life material as a way of avoiding bodywork, for example, or emotional work on what is going on in the here and now.

We have taken up birthing as an example of a much more general reality: the way in which our bodymind holds the memory of every crisis and transition in our lives, and constantly reinterprets each event in terms of every other event, creating clumps or clusters of imagery on the mental level which exist physically as organisations of tension in the muscles of the body. Accompanying these tension patterns are vivid and elaborate body-fantasies, which often emerge in the course of therapy.

For example, someone may experience themselves as being eaten up to the neck by a great snake-worm-monster – which is the body itself threatening to consume the ego-observer. Or they may experience their limbs as paralysed or amputated; they may sense a penis in their throat or rectum (which, again, is not necessarily a literal memory); they may feel as though they have a baby inside their womb or their chest, their head might balloon out to a vast size, or their whole body become minute; they may float off the ground or sink through it. Again, there may be vivid 'past life' experiences of torture or violent death. All of these are real examples from our clients or ourselves; all, however bizarre they may seem, are perfectly normal and healthy. This is the 'language' in which our bodymind unconscious 'thinks' and 'speaks'; often it needs to be explored in order to heal our wounds.

We want to close this rather brief survey with a very different form of 'primal pattern'. We have seen how the seed-form of a person's characteristic attitudes can be sought further and further back in their personal history – in birth, conception, and even previous lives (and we have questioned whether 'earlier' in this context means 'more basic'). But there is another form of pre-history which helps to shape our lives: the history of our family, and the characteristic themes and questions handed down and restated from generation to generation.

We cannot be sure of the mechanism by which we inherit our family themes. There is the obvious effect of childhood experiences, but there often seems to be something more fundamental, more mysterious, at work – 'inherited memory' inscribed in the cells themselves? Certainly it is not uncommon for someone to have a recurring issue or image in their life which relates directly to an experience, not of their own, but of a parent. In a very general sense we have inherited the unresolved issues of our parents' lives, issues which they may well have inherited from their parents, and so on back.

Through their upbringing, children will tend either to reproduce their parents' armouring – as when oppressive toilet training in her childhood leads a mother to be equally rigid with her children because she has internalised the need for rules; or else they will tend to react *against* the parental pattern – as when a father's thrusting character sets up a panicked crisis reaction in his child.

The parents' own patterns are a reproduction of or reaction to their own parents; with each generation a new synthesis is created from the new couple – who, of course, are attracted to each other partly by their corresponding character armour.

Yet couples are also attracted to each other by the intuitively sensed possibility of helping each other towards *healing*. However horrific the 'family theme', there is always the possibility of resolving it, of bringing it to an end, of bringing out its creative side. The extreme case is the family which abuses its children down through the generations, each child growing up to reproduce blindly its own agony. Even here it is as if the children are sent forth on their parents' behalf to try to do better; as if the parents are silently saying 'You do what we couldn't do; you bring this family process to a close.'

The same is true in the more ordinary and less horrific family situations, where there might be an inherited theme of guilt, or of struggling to 'better oneself', or of separation, or of sibling struggle.

Every family is a problem looking for a solution; every family member is an element in both the problem *and* the solution, elected to that role and usually unable to resign from it. And until the process is completed the issue will re-seed and reproduce itself – because that is the only way to avoid definitive failure. The very continuation of the family theme is a quest for its resolution, and this is the basis for hope in the family pattern which may otherwise seem utterly helpless, the individual bound hand and foot into a 'family curse'.

The set of patterns within which we as individuals live are rather like a hologram: each part contains within itself the whole, as the pattern-maker constantly re-synthesises our life story out of each new development.

Reichian work chooses to focus on the developmental phases of the first four or five years, knowing that this is not the whole story, that by the time we pass through these stages a great deal has already happened in our personal history and pre-history. We bring a lot of experience with us as we face these developmental thresholds, and this affects how we deal with them. Watching our own baby daughter, for instance, we have seen her manifest the whole sequence of phases within her first eighteen months.

What seems most important is the *sequence* – that wavelike streaming of energy down from the head to tail which repeats itself many times from conception to death just as it recurs constantly in the therapeutic process. It is relatively easy for a child to pass through a whole sequence in infancy, as our own daughter did, or even within the womb, without significant armouring being created.

What seems virtually impossible within our culture is for a child to pass the threshold of socialisation and gender, the 'Crisis' or 'Oedipal' stage, without being wounded. The nature of the child's response to this crisis, the style of armouring which she or he develops, will be decided by their *whole* history so far, by all the crises and challenges they have already faced.

Unless we meet with definite mishap, we may emerge from infancy with only minor scars to face the issues of gender identity and socialisation. It is how we deal with *these* issues, with the unnatural demands which society imposes on our 'original nature', that sets the seal on our approach to creativity, contact, openness, surrender.

11

Cosmic Streaming

> We are all struggling; none of us has gone far. Let your arrogance go, and look around inside.
>
> The blue sky opens out farther and farther, the daily sense of failure goes away, the damage I have done myself fades, the million suns come forward with light when I sit firmly in that world.
>
> I hear bells ringing that no one has shaken, inside 'love' there is more than we know of, rain pours down, although the sky is clear of clouds, there are whole rivers of light. The universe is shot through in all parts by a single sort of love. How hard it is to feel that joy in all our four bodies!
>
> Robert Bly, *The Kabir Book*

The work we have described opens people up to a whole range of new experiences, new and more intense emotions, new bodily sensations, new thoughts and understandings. It also opens us up, in many cases, to experiences which are generally referred to as 'psychic', 'spiritual' and 'supernatural'. Discovering these experiences through therapy helps us realise that such things are in fact profoundly *natural*, a part of our birthright walled off from us by the barrier of our armouring, sealed away in the distant, magical world of remembered childhood.

It would appear that as babies and children we do not suffer from the illusion of being totally separate beings. We exist as a particular 'place' or 'focus' in the field of existence; energy and desire sweep *through* us, move us, and move on. The 'spastic ego' develops partly in order to protect this wide-open quality from the madness, hate and pain we find around us – to create a walled garden in the desert of patriarchal culture.

The tragic paradox is that putting a wall around the garden also cuts it off from its sources of life. Separateness is itself an illusion, an insanity; the barriers we put up to defend our natural love and joyfulness also defend us against nature itself. Isolation preserves our sanity, but also drives us mad.

This is simply a restatement in more 'metaphysical' language of what we have been saying throughout the book. Life energy naturally *moves* – and our skin does not constitute a boundary to that movement. One of the forms that this streaming of energy takes is the human need and desire for contact: contact with other humans, with our own internal life, and with the natural world around us. But that natural world is much larger and fuller than our walled-off adult perceptions suggest.

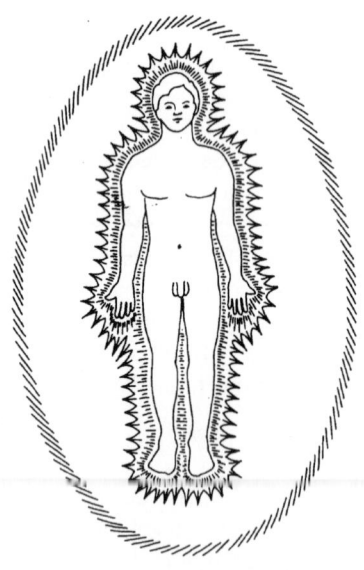

As we grow up, our perceptions are trained by what we are *expected* to see, hear and feel. When children show awareness of beings and forces which are invisible to the adults around them, those adults usually respond with fear ('there's something wrong with our child'), anger ('stop telling fibs') and incomprehension. As with sexuality, the child learns that this area of life is dangerous and not to be talked about In the long run, she usually learns *not* to see – and to half-forget that she ever could see.

When during therapy the armouring softens and starts to dissolve, so our barrier against the 'psychic' becomes softer and leakier; we begin to 'pick things up', to be more in touch with other people's thoughts and feelings, just as we are more in touch with our own. 'Picking things up' can happen in many other circumstances, especially with the use of certain drugs; some people do it all their lives. The focus on and trust in our own inner life which Reichian work develops will help dissolve intellectual assumptions about what we experience, and strengthen our grounded belief in what actually *does* happen.

Rather than keeping 'psychic' experiences in a separate compartment of life, either as 'fantasy' or 'special', we are able to integrate them with the rest of life.

This sphere of perception is in fact profoundly *ordinary*, an unacknowledged part of all human interaction. People can get into a real confusion of paranoia and self-importance if they fail to recognise this ordinariness, to recognise that 'extrasensory perception' flowers out of the five senses, and no authentic distinction can be drawn between the two any more than a line can be drawn on our neck to separate head from body.

All the great teaching systems explain that 'psychic powers' are essentially a side-effect of something else, which people often call 'spirituality'; the true realisation of the unity of all being. As it grows in us, not just as a head idea but as a *reality*, this knowledge brings up all our fear of deep contact. Psychics, spirituality, make us aware that we are not in fact separate beings, isolated egos in bags of skin. This is simultaneously a great joy and a great terror; the ego-illusion of separateness struggles to cling on, to save itself, to maintain the pretence.

You may notice a similarity between what we are saying here and our description in Chapters 4 and 6 of the eye segment and the Boundary character. It is when we are born that we have to face most starkly and brutally these issues of separation and openness. In the womb, the foetus is in a state of confluence with the mother's body; 'cosmic unity' is a bodily experience. At birth we must deal simultaneously with *isolation* – being cut off from our mother – and with *invasion* on sensory, physical and psychic levels. As we have said, Boundary characters, who are constantly dealing with these issues, are also often very sensitive to energy and to psychic phenomena. Because they tend also to be ungrounded, however, separate from their own bodies and terrified of invasion, their perception of psychic events tends to be confused and mixed with fantasy and paranoia.

The boundary position in each of us reacts in a similar way to the realisation of unity: it seeks to protect its barriers. There is the danger of what Chögyam Trungpa calls 'spiritual materialism' – an empty parody of genuine openness in which the ego is secretly congratulating itself on having 'let go of the ego'. It is fearfully easy either to become puffed up with your incredible psychic talent, or else to give the whole thing away to 'God' or to some guru in a pompous and insipid religiosity, which is a defence against the simple here-and-now reality.

Both giving and receiving therapy seem to us forms of active meditation. They are about constantly letting go, constantly coming back to the core, to simplicity, to what is. For both of us there is a special sense of connection with Buddhism, in particular with Tibetan Vajrayana Buddhism and its roots in shamanic tradition.

Shamanism is the archaic psychic tradition of our planet, which survives in essentially similar forms in many tribal cultures. With its focus on the body, on symbolic death and rebirth processes, on energy, on transformation, Reichian therapy is a thoroughly shamanic form of healing. As we go on with the work, it is sometimes as if we are discovering and re-owning all the ancient healing traditions of the world.

This was very much what happened to Reich himself – though he unfortunately lacked the background knowledge to realise it. Following through his clear and honest perceptions of energy in nature, he ended up totally out on a limb as far as 1950s Western culture was concerned; a true witch doctor, creating rain, distributing magical objects, exorcising, and alchemically processing exotic substances. Tragically, he went on insisting that his work was 'scientific', appealing for recognition from a scientific community which was hostile to everything he represented.

What we can most easily relate to in Reich's later explorations is his emphasis on the unity of nature and on our role as natural beings. He had a tremendous vision of the streaming of energy in the cosmos, the galaxies, the oceans, the weather – and in our own bodies. He saw it as the same energy, following the same patterns, the same dance. Although Reich condemned 'mysticism' – by which he meant flight from bodily reality – his own vision is in the best sense a truly mystical one.

Yet it is also highly concrete, and grew out of some very real and functional discoveries. 'Orgone' is not simply some vaguely uplifting notion, but an energy that can be directly *felt* by anyone who takes the trouble.

The simplest form of orgone device consists of several alternating layers of wool (such as an old blanket – not synthetic) and steel wool (the sort of stuff brillo pads are made of, obtainable from most hardware shops). This multi-layer sandwich is enclosed, for convenience, in a thin cotton cushion-cover. You will find that a distinct energy emanates from the top layer of steel wool; experienced by many people as warmth and tingling, it takes a few minutes to build up if you sit on the cushion or put your hand on it, a sensation which develops into a sense of 'fullness' and a natural desire to move away from the cushion.

Many people have to train themselves to recognise orgone, but once we tune in to it the sensation is very recognisable – and closely akin to feelings we have during bodywork sessions. This is a natural life energy, which the cushion concentrates rather than creates. Children often sense the energy immediately, since they have no reason to think there's anything odd about it.

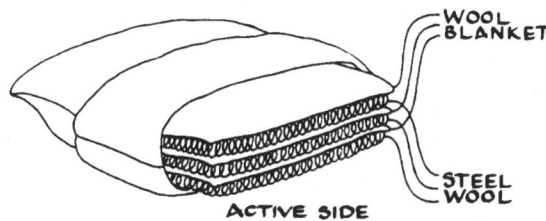

Orgone energy in this form – a simple 'orgone accumulator' – charges up an organism. It is useful for states of exhaustion and lowness, the sort of time when we're vulnerable to colds and flu, and its use helps cuts, burns and so on to heal faster. *Don't take our word for it* – try it for yourself! Note that someone who is already *over*charged will probably get a headache or other unpleasant effects from using the cushion. It shouldn't be applied to sensitive areas like head and heart for more than a few minutes, and when not in use it should be kept with the 'active' (steel wool) side face down or folded in on itself. Do not use the accumulator around colour TV, strip lighting, etc. – it will also concentrate this sort of energy.

The accumulator works much better, and produces a more pleasant feeling, on clear, fresh, blue-sky days, since it condenses and concentrates the energy which is in the atmosphere already. If the weather is oppressive and polluted, then so is the orgone energy. This is how Reich was led into working directly on the weather with other orgone devices – the 'cloudbuster' as he rather unfortunately named it, which we would prefer to call a 'cloudmelter'. This implausible Buck Rogers mechanism, according to all the available evidence, actually works ...

We don't want to be drawn too far into the wonders of orgone physics, but we do want to make it clear that devices like this, unlike orthodox Western technology, cannot be separated from the feeling state of the people using them. In order to work effectively with the weather, a person needs to be in a sufficiently clear and open state to *contact* the condition of the atmosphere, to perceive how blocked or mobile it is – in fact, to give it a therapy session!

It seems to us that orgone may be not so much *the* life energy as a particular form of life energy. As Reich describes it, and as we ourselves experience it, orgone has some quite specific characteristics. It has a special relationship with water, which is why it links with water vapour in the atmosphere, and also why it 'streams', 'pools', 'condenses' and so on. It flows along the length of the human body, and is deeply bound up with orgasm. Other world traditions describe other types of life energy with properties which are similar but *not* identical: 'prana', 'chi' and so on cannot simply be identified with orgone, or with each other.

Similarly, just because many of the great healing systems describe energy centres in roughly the same areas of the body, it is not right to claim that they are all the same. The numbers, positions and descriptions of 'chakras' (a term from the yogic system only) can vary quite considerably. At the same time, though, it is rather striking how closely our system of *segments* parallels the yogic system of *chakras*.

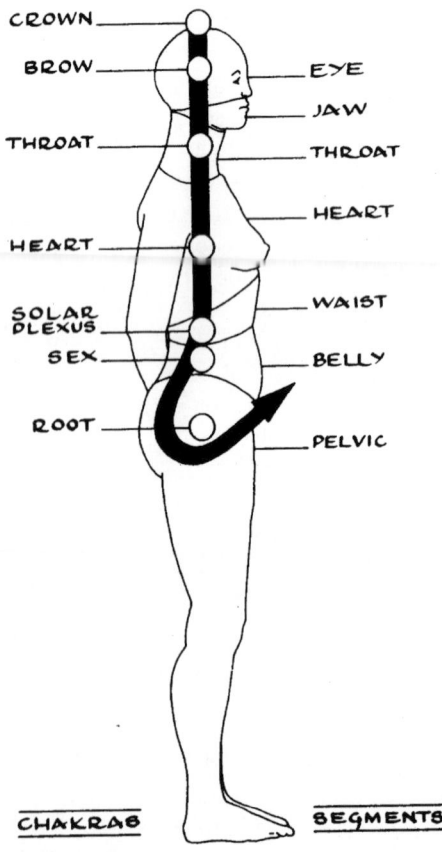

Using Reichian work there are many other ways in which we re-contact concepts and experiences which are a familiar part of esoteric systems from around the world. We start to perceive and to work with the aura – the energy field surrounding the physical body, which is often more easily sensed in the hands than seen with the eyes. We become sensitive to earth energy, the force used by dowsers and the builders of stone circles and other ancient sacred sites. Many of these have an energy that is very reminiscent of orgone, and some at least are built on a similar principle of 'layering'. From Reichian therapy we can move in all sorts of directions into a new, rich universe.

We must however emphasise the *difference* of Reichian work, with its stress on being grounded in our own immediate experience, and in the reality of the body, from most esoteric, psychic and spiritual groupings. It is perilously easy even for experienced Reichians to 'take flight', to soar off into ungrounded fantasies and delusions as a means of avoiding the anxiety of authentic contact. Reich himself, in the last years of his life, seems to some extent to have lost touch with the commonsense ordinariness of life. It's also very easy to enter into a passionately enthusiastic transference relationship with some teacher or guru which you would never be able to leave unexamined with your therapist!

The teaching systems of the East in particular seem to rely on and use the positive transference relationship between disciple and guru as a means to an end, building up an intensity of need and fear which finally enables the disciple to break through to another level of understanding. This process may well have a positive outcome when properly carried out, but such worship and surrender is clearly open to profound abuse in the hands of a teacher whose own selfish ego, whose own character blocks, are still in command.

Seen from the more metaphysical viewpoint that we are using in this chapter, the underlying theme of the work we do is *embodiment*: choosing to be here, to be a body, with all the painful awkwardness and recalcitrance of the physical world. As we have said, it is often at birth that we most brutally face the pain of embodiment, and may wish – and try – not to be here. But embodiment is not something we do only once in life – it is a commitment that must be renewed over and over again as each crisis and challenge encourages us to retreat from life, to take refuge in illusions and fantasies.

Connection with the cosmos is not a matter of floating off into visions, but of engaging with the joy and beauty of the real world – making our visions into reality. We have each chosen to be here; and our 'mission' seems to be to do with incarnating as much as possible of the beauty we can sense and imagine. Human beings are like trees, rooted in the ground, branches reaching up into the sky, trunk joining the two into a unity. Some people need to be anchored more strongly in the physical world; others need to be 'lifted' into greater awareness of the subtle, spiritual dimension of life. The goal is always ultimate wholeness.

Entering into this therapy doesn't commit you to believing in fairies and flying saucers! The work helps to put each person more in touch with their own authentic experience, enabling them at every point to *test out* what they are told, and what they seem to perceive, to an extent which is unusual in our brainwashed and beglamoured society. Letting go of compulsive defences, letting go of the cloud of anxiety which usually stands between us and the world, allows each of us to make our own choices about what to believe and what to explore.

12

Connections and Directions

> To remain whole, be twisted!
> To become straight, let yourself be bent.
> To become full, be hollow.
> Be tattered, that you may be renewed.
> Those that have little, may get more.
> Those that have much, are but perplexed.
> Therefore the Sage
> Clasps the Primal Unity.
>
> Lao Tsu, *Tao Te Ching*

The style of working with people which we have described is a form of psychotherapy; it is also, as we have tried to make clear, a political and a spiritual practice; but above all, we see it as a form of *healing*, linked with the many methods and techniques being discovered and rediscovered at the present time as part of the 'alternative healing', 'alternative medicine' movement. We very much identify with that movement, and see our work as within the great stream of human energy, going back to the Old Stone Age, which understands healing as something done with humans rather than with illnesses, a process of *making whole* rather than the elimination of troublesome symptoms.

It is time to explain how we see our work within the whole web of healing and therapeutic practices; which approaches are our natural allies and complements; to explore some possible lines of distinction and disagreement; and to clarify how we see our own potential contribution to the practice of healing.

It seems to us that healing takes place essentially through a *relationship*. The relationship is often primarily that between client and healer, which comes to stand for the relationship between the client and the world. This is the process which we have described in Chapter 8 as 'transference', and we believe that it arises in every form of healing work. Healing strongly encourages 'parent–child' interactions: I am coming to you for help, asking you to kiss it better, to feed me, to look after me, with all the positive and negative feelings that stirs up in me, all the love and the rebellion. Equally, this will stir up in you all sorts of positive and negative parental feelings about me.

As we have argued in Chapter 8, these feelings can be an obstacle to the healing process, but more deeply, they are a unique opportunity to examine the issues at the heart of the client's problem – their feelings about power, dependency, safety, embodiment itself. A healer who cannot or will not recognise and work with these issues of relationship is severely handicapped. It will be hard for them to see clearly what is going on in the healing process, the underlying transactions behind the surface. They will find it difficult to understand why some clients 'get better' and others don't, and what their *own* needs and demands are doing to the healing work.

The theory of transference comes out of the Freudian roots of Reichian therapy, and it is still possible to understand what we do as a form of psychoanalysis – though a very mutated form. Our concern is still with the unconscious memories of childhood traumas and the unconscious structures of defence which they have created. The role of breathing in Reichian work is, in one way, very similar to the role of free association in classical analysis, the analyst says 'just say whatever comes up' and watches the blocks to this process, while the Reichian says 'just breathe freely' and watches the blocks to *this* process.

Within the range of psychotherapies, however, we would identify at least as strongly with the cluster of styles and practices known as 'humanistic psychology'. Some of the differences between this and classical psychoanalysis are an emphasis on the client's own responsibility and empowerment; an attitude of 'whatever works' rather than strictly defined techniques; and a focus on the 'here and now' rather than on past history. This last theme is identified most often with Gestalt Therapy: it is very much a position we share – that there will always be more to uncover about the past, always more old pain to 'get out', and that the real healing comes from absorbing the past and moving on.

The influences here work both ways. The whole of humanistic psychology has been very much influenced by Reich's work, so that in a sense our fusion of the two represents 'what Reich might have done if he had lived into the 1980s'. Or so we would like to think! In practice, Reich was very much committed to the idea of the therapist-as-expert, and even believed that only medical doctors should give therapy. In any case, the influence is strong; Fritz Perls, founder of Gestalt, in particular, derived more of his ideas than are generally realised from Reich's work – and we in turn use several of Perls' techniques.

This 'here-and-now' emphasis is the mental and verbal expression of what we have described as the theme of *embodiment*. It is through *bodywork – when they are open to it –* that a person can most strongly confront, and change, their resistance to being here and now, can make a new commitment to facing and resolving the problems of life. Although we may quite often not touch a person during a therapy session, or even directly engage with their body life, it is always a crucial foundation to the work we do. We feel that purely verbal therapies are handicapped in facilitating deep change.

There are many forms of bodywork available these days, and although Reich was the first person to link bodywork into psychotherapy many people have since independently made the same breakthrough. There are also several schools of bodywork directly descended from Reich's work apart from our own – historically speaking they are our cousins. These schools often refer to themselves, or are referred to by others, as 'neo-Reichian'. We'd like to say a little bit about two of these: Bioenergetics and Postural Integration.

Bioenergetics, developed by Alexander Lowen (a therapist of immense wisdom and love who studied with and received therapy from Reich), is in some ways very close to our own work. Some important differences are that Bioenergetics focuses more on a standing, 'vertically grounded' position rather than a lying down, 'horizontally grounded' one, and that it works more with postures and exercises than with direct touch. Both of these features put an emphasis on qualities of independence, assertiveness and control, rather than on surrender and acceptance, so that Bioenergetics will perhaps be ideal for different clients than those who like our method of work.

Postural Integration is a deep restructuring of the body's connective tissue which surrounds each muscle and muscle group: it believes that until the connective tissue is made supple and flexible it is not physically possible for muscles to relax and lengthen. Postural Integration is profoundly influenced by Reichian ways of seeing, and emphasises the role of the breath and of armouring.

A big difference between our work and Postural Integration – and even more so with Rolfing, another form of deep massage restructuring – is that we try very hard to avoid a concept of how someone *should* be: to avoid offering a model, either implicit or explicit – of how a person *ought* to breathe, *ought* to stand, *ought* to move. In practice, of course, the difference is only one of emphasis; we do inevitably have a very strong sense of the difference between health and unhealth, while conversely any good practitioner respects the uniqueness of each individual.

There is, however, a big difference between the programmatic approach of an essentially *remedial* system like Postural Integration, and our work's focus on opening up to our own core, to our innate capacity for growth and healing. In bodywork just as on other levels, we trust the unconscious wisdom of the individual, and its capacity to find the right path if our ego 'gets out of the way'.

What in practice happens, in the course of therapy – what has happened many times to each of us – is that we begin to experience an *inner* sense of 'not being right' in our bodies. We sense a *need* to be helped in expanding, lengthening, straightening, softening. This, it seems to us, is the point at which it is fruitful to find a remedial practitioner of one sort or another, the point at which our bodymind is ready and able to accept and use this new way of holding ourselves, rather than immediately 'snapping back' into the old shape. Without emotional change, physical change won't stick; equally, without physical change emotional change won't stick.

We have discovered some forms of remedial work which are tremendously gentle and subtle in style, encouraging and allowing growth rather than pushing the individual. The Alexander Technique is a non-invasive approach to opening us out into a more natural and relaxed posture, an effortless way of being in the world; in many ways it seems the perfect complement to Reichian work, approaching the same goals from the opposite direction. It may well be that Alexander practitioners also have something to learn from a therapy which involves emotional release. T'ai Chi, though not a therapy (and indeed the Alexander Technique doesn't see itself as a therapy), is another gentle and enormously powerful way of aligning us with subtle energy flows, teaching us to make less and less effort to achieve better and better results. And the Feldenkrais Method seems to be a third, independent style of working with the same principles of non-effort, not-doing, going with the flow.

If we feel slightly cautious about remedial bodywork, which in some of its forms can simply introduce a whole new lot of tensions to cover up and mask the original ones, then we feel a lot more dubious about methods of 'remedial mindwork'. By this we mean all the vast range of therapies and 'positive thinking' techniques which aim to alter our thoughts and behaviour to match a conscious ideal.

The most obvious example of this is Cognitive Behavioural Therapy (CBT), a set of techniques which in skilful hands can be highly effective in removing symptoms like phobias, compulsions, blushing, and so on. Certainly, such methods are a lot less harmful than alternatives like drugging or ECT, but we are convinced that what is going on here is *masking*, a suppression of symptoms rather than working with the problem which those symptoms *express*. Just as allopathic medicine, by suppressing the symptoms of a deep problem, can make it harder and harder for the body to heal itself, so CBT can make it harder and harder for real emotional healing to take place. (More recent developments in CBT recognise and try to address this limitation.)

There are other versions of behaviour modification with a very different image and appearance; these work with affirmations, with visualisation, with positive thinking. Most of these techniques assert that 'we create our own reality'. There is very deep truth in this statement, but there is also often a very superficial illusion. We *can* create our own reality (so long as it conforms sufficiently with the universe's reality); we can identify and let go of the negative 'scripts' and assumptions through which we constantly recreate our own suffering. But we can also impose a layer of illusion *on top of* an inner negativity, a quite false and unlived positivity which is the mental equivalent of a new layer of physical tensions masking the original problem.

What all these systems have in common is a tinkering approach to the human unconscious, seeing it as a box of tricks where one has only to press the right button, to find the right switch, in order to achieve the desired goal. The bodymind unconscious actually knows better than our conscious mind; it is the source of our wisdom and the source of our life. Physical or emotional symptoms of dis-ease are messages that our conscious behaviour is out of balance, and that we need to return to the source – not to find some simple and effortless way of *pretending* to feel better.

We are not saying, of course, that all work with affirmations and positive visualisation is damaging. In fact, we use these techniques ourselves. But what is vital is to check out our response to the new message o*n all levels*; never to suppress an inner resistance or denial, but to give it all the space it needs to express and discharge itself. As with remedial bodywork, such techniques are only healing when the emotional space exists to make use of them.

The idea of *space* seems to come up over and over again in our work: the need to create and allow a physical, emotional, mental, spiritual spaciousness in which we can let things be, let ourselves be, rather than trying to tinker all the time. The need for real change, both in ourselves and in the world, can then flower out of space and quietness.

Apart from the specifically 'neo-Reichian' approaches, one form of growth work with which we feel a special connection is Rebirthing, or 'conscious connected breathing', which is centred on a simple and powerful bodily technique: encouraging clients to breathe continuously in and out with no break between breaths, focusing high in the chest, and keeping breathing no matter what feelings and thoughts come up. This is an amazingly powerful technique, highly effective in many ways in releasing blocks and coming through to joyous, streaming sensations and spacious attitudes.

Rebirthers combine conscious connected breathing with a quite elaborate set of *ideas* about which we are less enthusiastic, and which seem in many ways quite separate from the breathing technique itself. It is as if Rebirthing has become a sort of grab-bag of whatever notions and methods its founders and developers have come across, simply throwing them all together rather than incorporating new ideas around the central theme. The breathing technique itself, however, is very valuable, and we sometimes incorporate it into our own work. It brings people into contact with their core resistances very quickly, and also into contact with their core of health. In fact it is a way of breathing which often happens spontaneously, a deeply natural way of releasing trauma that one can often see in small babies and in animals. Our own daughter seemed to 'clear' the effects of her birth by repeatedly Rebirthing herself in the first months of life.

We would also like to mention Polarity Therapy, an approach based on Indian Ayurvedic medicine, which combines bodywork, energy balancing, nutrition and psychotherapy in a complex and powerful synthesis. From our own experience of receiving Polarity sessions, it is working with the same body energy as Reichian therapy – though there are differences in how this energy is understood.

In relating our own approach to other healing and therapeutic techniques we find that in some cases we can pick up and use elements of other approaches, adapting them to our own needs. In other cases a healing system feels more self-contained, as if one either has to work within that worldview or leave it be – thus we might recommend a client to go off and work with another practitioner, either temporarily or indefinitely.

To some extent we are increasingly moving away from the 'Reichian' label, as our work, while still in tune with Reich's essential vision of the world, becomes less and less like anything he himself did. We have to take on, as well, the fact that Reich himself came to despair of the effectiveness of individual therapy, saying that a twisted tree cannot be straightened, and that the only hope was to work with infants and with the orgone energy systems of the atmosphere.

It is true that a twisted tree cannot be straightened; it is true also that a human being can never have their past experiences *erased*, nor the imprint of those experiences on their bodymind. But this does not strike us as a cause for despair. Sometimes we feel like despairing – as must everyone who has any sensitivity to what is happening in the world. But even a twisted tree can thrive and blossom, can take joy and heart in its own strength and survival, and can send forth seedlings with the chance of growing straighter and more joyfully still. This assumes that straightness is in the nature of the tree; and maybe humans are more like hawthorns, whose grace is in their twistedness as it reflects the elemental forces which have shaped them.

Individual therapy and healing, as well as having intrinsic value, are contributions to the great work of healing our planet, and healing our relationship with our planet. How can we free our energies enough to work effectively at this daunting project?

This book constitutes one possible answer to that question. A part of dealing with our despair about the planet's future, as Joanna Macy has argued, is to face that despair, to reach down into the grief and fear, to reach through to the underlying wellsprings of creative action. There are profound connections between our feelings about the planet and our feelings about our individual history. If we are sensitive to the poisoning of the biosphere, is this because it resonates with the poisoning of our own feelings and energy? If we fear explosion and destruction, is this connected with fear of our own repressed anger and excitement?

These are real objective threats, and it is precisely in order to be able to face them that we need to look at our own material. In fact, we can even understand the great arsenals of potential annihilation as themselves the *result* of armouring, of repression – human orgasmic energy, with its secondary violence and hatefulness, all exported and projected into The Bomb, because we cannot acknowledge and befriend these forces within ourselves.

Thus growth work can be a force for good in the wider world, as well as in the individual interaction of client and therapist. But it can also be a force for evil. There are many techniques discovered or rediscovered by figures in the 'growth movement' which are powerfully effective in changing people's attitudes and behaviour, but which are in themselves value-free, equally effective in producing almost *any* sort of change. The transference relationship can become discipleship; the crisis and surrender which can be profoundly healing can also be the collapse and self-loss of brainwashing.

Many therapies, and not just the dramatic cultish ones, are devoted to brainwashing. They see their role as one of 'normalisation', turning their clients and patients back into ordinary, passive members of society who will then play by the accepted rules, even if those rules are destructive to life and creativity.

With any growth technique it is right and sensible to ask: What is your vision? How do you see human beings, and their place in nature? What sort of society do you want to live in, and how do you want to move towards it? A large number of growth practitioners, it seems, are unable or unwilling to answer these fundamental questions. In this book, as well as trying to share our techniques and insights, we have attempted to offer *our* answers.

Further Reading

This is only a small selection of possible literature: the bibliographies in some of the books by and about Reich will give you further directions. Unfortunately some of the best books are out of print, and you may have to search for them on the Internet; often there are several editions.

Works listed in relation to one chapter will often be relevant to other chapters as well. But each book is usually only mentioned once; however any book that is actually quoted from will be listed in relation to each chapter where it appears, with the relevant page reference.

INTRODUCTION TO THE SECOND EDITION

On state regulation of therapy:
- *Regulating the Psychological Therapies: From taxonomy to taxidermy,* Denis Postle (Ross-on-Wye: PCCS Books, 2007)

- *Implausible Professions: Arguments for pluralism and autonomy in psychotherapy and counselling,* Richard House and Nick Totton, eds (Ross-on-Wye: PCCS Books, 1997)

On attachment:
- *Attachment,* John Bowlby (London: Pelican, 1969)
- *The Search for the Secure Base: Attachment theory and psychotherapy,* Jeremy Holmes (London: Brunner-Routledge, 2001)

On attachment theory, trauma and neuroscience:
- *Why Love Matters: How affection shapes a baby's brain,* Sue Gerhardt (Hove: Routledge, 2004)

On trauma:
- See Further Reading for Chapter 2

The quotation from Reich about 'contact with the world' is from:

- *Character Analysis* (New York: Farrar, Straus and Giroux, 1972), p. 271. In the same book he discusses the 'genital character' on pages 176ff.

Nick's collected poems:
- *Press When Illuminated: New and selected poems, 1968 – 2003,* Nick Totton (Cambridge: Salt, 2004)

On Hakomi:
- *Body-Centered Psychotherapy: The Hakomi Method,* Ron Kurtz (Mendocino, CA: LifeRhythm, 2007)

On Authentic Movement:
- *Offering from the Conscious Body: The discipline of Authentic Movement,* Janet Adler (Rochester, VT: Bear & Co, 2002)

- *Authentic Movement,* 2 vols, Patriazia Pallaro, ed (London: Jessica Kingsley, 1999 and 2007)

On Process Work:
- A book which covers both theory and practice is *Riding the Horse Backwards,* Arnold Mindell and Amy Mindell (London: Arkana, 1992).

CHAPTER 1: CONTEXTS

The two major biographies of Reich – both by practising therapists – are:
- *Fury on Earth,* Myron Sharaf (London: Hutchinson, 1983)

- *Wilhelm Reich: His life and work,* David Boadella (London: Arkana, 1988)

Also useful on Reich:
- *Reich for Beginners,* David Zane Mairowitz and German Gonzalez (London: Writers and Readers, 1986)
A cartoon account, enjoyable and essentially accurate, leaning over backwards to be fair even against the authors' own beliefs.

- *A Book of Dreams,* Peter Reich (London: Picador, 1974)
A strange, moving account by Reich's son of life with him in his last years, and then of dealing with his death.

- *I'm a Doctor on an Expedition,* Heidrun Mossner (DVD, 2003)
A video portrait of Reich's daughter, Eva, who carried on much of his work, in old age.

Further Reading 151

On Reich's work and ideas:
- *Selected Writings*, Wilhelm Reich (New York: Farrar, Straus and Giroux, 1961)

- *Melting Armour*, William West (self-published, available from 12 Torbay Rd, Manchester M12 8XD, England). A pamphlet outlining the style of work we look at in this book, intended to help people exchange sessions.

- *Wilhelm Reich and Orgonomy*, Ola Raknes (Baltimore, MD: Pelican, 1971)

- *Wilhelm Reich: Psychoanalyst and radical naturalist*, Robert S Corrington (New York: Farrar, Straus and Giroux, 2003)

On Reich's origins in psychoanalysis:
- *The Water in the Glass: Body and mind in psychoanalysis*, Nick Totton (London: Rebus Press/Karnac, 1998)

CHAPTER 2: ENERGY AND ARMOUR

- *Orgone, Reich and Eros: Wilhelm Reich's Theory of Life Energy*, William Mann (New York: Simon and Schuster, 1973)

- *The Function of the Orgasm*, Wilhelm Reich (London: Souvenir Press, 1989)
Reich's own intellectual autobiography, charting the development of his work up to the mid-1940s, and giving a relatively readable account of his central ideas.

Three explorations of energy and armour by leading 'neo-Reichian' therapists:
- *Bioenergetics*, Alexander Lowen (London: Arkana, 1994)

- *Emotional Anatomy*, Stanley Keleman (Berkeley, CA: Center Press, 1985)

- *Lifestreams: An introduction to Biosynthesis*, David Boadella (London: Routledge and Kegan Paul, 1987)

- *Freud for Beginners*, Richard Appignanesi and Oscar Zarate (London: Icon Books, 1994)

Freud on the ego:
- 'The Ego and the Id', in *On Metapsychology*, Sigmund Freud (Penguin Freud Library Vol 11; London: Penguin, 1984), and in other editions of Freud's works.

- *Children of the Future*, Wilhelm Reich (New York: Farrar, Straus and Giroux, 1983)
This brings together all Reich's writings about armouring in infants and children.

Illness and emotion:
- *A Rose to a Sick Friend: A positive way to approach your illness*, Tessa Goldhawk (Bath: Gateway Books, 1989)

- *You Can Heal Your Life*, Louise Hay (Hay House, 2004) – approach this with caution and a pinch of salt!

On trauma, three of the most useful books are:
- *Waking the Tiger: Healing trauma*, Peter Levine (Berkeley, CA: North Atlantic Books, 1997)

- *The Body Remembers Casebook*, Babette Rothschild (New York: Norton, 2003)

- *Trauma and the Body*, Pat Ogdon, Kekuni Minton and Clare Pain (New York: Norton, 2006)

CHAPTER 3: SURRENDER

For a Reichian approach to flaccid muscles alongside rigid ones, which are usually emphasised more, see detailed information at: http://www.bodynamicusa.com/AboutBDYN.html and also some of the articles in:
- *Body, Breath and Consciousness: A Somatics anthology*, Ian Macnaughton, ed (Berkeley, CA: North Atlantic Books, 2004)

- *Thoughts Without a Thinker: Psychotherapy from a Buddhist perspective*, Mark Epstein (Duckworth, 1997)

- *Cutting Through Spiritual Materialism*, Chögyam Trungpa Rinpoche (Boston: Shambhala, 1987)

- *How to Change Yourself and Your World: A manual of co-counselling theory and practice*, Rose Evison and Richard Horobin (Sheffield: Co-Counselling Phoenix, 1991)

- *Sexuality: A biopsychosocial approach*, Chess Denman (London: Palgrave, 2004)

Further Reading   153

CHAPTER 4: THE SEGMENTS

• *Man in the Trap: The causes of blocked sexual energy*, Elsworth F Baker (New York: Collier Macmillan, 1967)
This is a highly orthodox Reichian work, and while we don't agree with everything Baker says, he gives a very thorough account of the segments and other aspects of Reich's theory.

Some books about the neuroscientific findings that support these ideas:
• *Descartes' Error: Emotion, reason and the human brain*, Antonio Damasio (New York: Vintage, 2006)

• *The Feeling of What Happens: Body, emotion and the making of consciousness*, Antonio Damasio (New York: Vintage, 2000)

• *Molecules of Emotion: Why you feel the way you feel*, Candace Pert (New York: Pocket Books, 1999)

Two examples from the wide range of books available on body-patterning, each giving a similar but somewhat different version of the segments:
• *The Body Reveals*, Ron Kurtz and Hector Prestera (San Francisco: HarperSanFrancisco, 1991)

• *Bodymind*, Ken Dychtwald (New York: Tarchor, 1000)

And some books which are informative about specific segments, although mostly not using Reichian ideas:
• *Better Eyesight without Glasses*, WH Bates (London: Grafton, 1989)
A marvellous classic relating physical/emotional/spiritual aspects of vision.

• *Body Learning: An introduction to the Alexander Technique*, Michael Gelb (London: Aurum Press, 2004)
One of several good books available on the technique, which particularly illuminates the head/neck/back relationship.

• *The Way to Vibrant Health*, Alexander Lowen and Leslie Lowen (Alachua, FL: Bioenergetics Press, 2003)
A collection of body exercises based on neo-Reichian principles.

The quotation about 'the genuine heart of sadness' is from:
• *Shambhala*, Chögyam Trungpa Rinpoche (Shambhala), p. 45. This book has wise things to say about several of the segments we are discussing.

- *The Endless Web: Fascial anatomy and physical reality*, R Louis Schultz and Rosemary Feitis (Berkeley, CA: North Atlantic Books, 1996)
A book about Rolfing, which gives detailed and fascinating information about the body, casting a lot of light on the segments discussed here.

If you like working with the sort of exercises we offer in this chapter, then we recommend:
- *The Way to Vibrant Health: A manual of Bioenergetic exercises*, Alexander Lowen and Leslie Lowen (New York: Harper Colophon, 1977)

Grounding, centering and facing:
- *Lifestreams: An introduction to Biosynthesis*, David Boadella (London: Routledge and Kegan Paul, 1987), Chapter 2 onwards

The quotation starting 'if our relationship with the ground is tenuous' is from:
- *The Human Ground: Sexuality, self and survival*, Stanley Keleman (Berkeley, CA: Center Press, 1981)

CHAPTER 5: GROWING UP

Probably the best material on these themes is in novels, stories, poems and films, especially about childhood and adolescence. A few examples out of many:
- *The Waves*, Virginia Woolf (many editions available)

- *The Prelude*, William Wordsworth (many editions)

- *Oranges Are Not the Only Fruit*, Jeannette Winterson (London: Bloomsbury, 1991) and the TV version

- *Brokeback Mountain*, Annie Proulx (London: Fourth Estate, 1991) and the film version

- *Hideous Kinky,* Emma Freud (London: Penguin, 1993) and the film version

- *Frankie and Stanky*, Barbara Trapido (London: Bloomsbury, 2004)

- *The Summer Book*, Tove Jansson (London: Sort of Books, 2003)

- *My So-Called Life,* TV series available on DVD

- *Little Miss Sunshine*, DVD

The novels of Jacqueline Wilson, Anne Fine, and many other children's writers.

By far the best non-fiction book we know on infancy, and one which is very exciting from a Reichian point of view, is:
- *The Interpersonal World of the Infant*, Daniel N Stern (New York: Basic Books, 1985)

And a more accessible account of similar material:
- *Diary of a Baby: What your child sees, feels and experiences*, Daniel N Stern (New York: Basic Books, 1992)

Two helpful books about children's experience:
- *The Child's Discovery of the Mind*, Janet Wilde Astington (Cambridge, MA: Harvard University Press, 1993)

- *Children's Minds*, Margaret Donaldson (New York: HarperCollins, 1986)

We have also learned a lot about childhood from the psychoanalytic ideas of DW Winnicott; for an introduction, try:
- *Winnicott*, Adam Phillips (London: Fontana Modern Masters, 1988)

Another highly stimulating therapy text, although we disagree with some of its stances, is:
- *The Road Less Travelled*, M Scott Peck (London: Rider, 1985)

Reich discusses the three layers of personality in:
- *The Mass Psychology of Fascism* (Harmondsworth: Penguin, 1975), pp 13–14

For a wonderful account of embryonic and foetal development, see:
- *Embryogenesis*, Richard Grossinger (Berkeley, CA: North Atlantic Books, 1986)

CHAPTERS 6 AND 7: CHARACTER

- *Character Analysis*, Wilhelm Reich (New York: Farrar, Straus and Giroux, 1980)

- *Body-Centred Psychotherapy: The Hakomi Method*, Ron Kurtz (Mendocino, CA: LifeRhythm, 1990)

There is a far more detailed account of character in the earlier version of this book, now only obtainable second hand and with difficulty:
- *Hakomi Therapy,* Ron Kurtz (Boulder, CO: Hakomi Institute, 1985)

- *The Language of the Body: Physical dynamics of character structure*, Alexander Lowen (Alachua, FL: Bioenergetics Press, 2006)

- *Characterological Transformation*, Stephen M Johnson (New York: Norton, 1985)
In this and several other volumes, Johnson offers a synthesis of character theory and American ego psychology. We strongly disagree with some of his positions, but this is probably the most extensive account of character yet produced.

There is a chapter on Reichian character theory, alongside other ideas about different styles of personhood, in:
- *Character and Personality Types*, Nick Totton and Michael Jacobs (Maidenhead: Open University Press, 2001)

- *The Divided Self*, RD Laing (Harmondsworth: Penguin, 1965)

CHAPTER 8: THERAPY

There are fascinating case histories and accounts of therapeutic work in all of the books listed by Reich himself.

Two books of Nick's:
- *Body Psychotherapy: An introduction* (Maidenhead: Open University Press, 2003)
A survey of the field with some specific ideas of my own.

- *New Dimensions in Body Psychotherapy* (Maidenhead: Open University Press, 2005)
A collection of chapters by practitioners of different styles, including a chapter on Embodied-Relational Therapy, the latest incarnation of the work we describe in this book.

Some of the best books we know on different varieties of body psychotherapy:
- *Emotional First Aid*, Sean Haldane (Barrytown, NY: Station Hill, 1988)
A simple, practical crystallisation of body-based emotional discharge techniques, unfortunately very hard to find.

- *The Anatomy of Change*, Richard Heckler (Boston: Shambhala, 1984)
A classic work which combines martial arts and Reichian perspectives.

- *The Body in Recovery*, John Conger (Berkeley, CA: Frog Ltd, 1994)
A good, eloquent book on a version of Reichian work fairly similar to our own.

- *Body-Mind Psychotherapy*, Susan Aposhyan (New York: Norton, 2004)

Further Reading

An excellent account of the 21st century version of body psychotherapy, strongly grounded in neuroscience.
* *Body of Awareness: A somatic and developmental approach to psychotherapy*, Ruella Frank (Cambridge, MA: Gestalt Press/Analytic Press, 2001)
A movement-oriented account with roots in Gestalt.

As accounts of Reichian therapy or of the therapeutic process in general we recommend:
* *Other Women*, Lisa Alther (Harmondsworth: Penguin, 1986)
A novel about one woman's therapy, switching between the client's and the therapist's viewpoints.

* *Me and the Orgone*, Orson Bean (London: St Martin's Press, 1977)
A very funny account of one person's experience of classical Reichian therapy.

* *Reich, Jung, Regardie and Me: The unhealed healer*, J Marvin Spiegelman (Scottsdale, AZ: New Falcon, 1992)
An eminent Jungian analyst describes his experience of Reichian therapy.

* *Working with the Dreaming Body*, Arnold Mindell (Portland, OR: Lao Tse Press, 2006)
A very different approach which has nonetheless influenced us a great deal – Process Oriented Psychotherapy.

* *In Search of a Therapist*, edited by Michael Jacobs and Moira Walker (Milton Keynes: Open University Press, 1995)
A series of five books, in each of which six therapists from different disciplines explain how they would work with the same client.

CHAPTER 9: POWER

On 'power-for' and 'power-over':
* *The Other Side of Power*, Claude Steiner (New York: Grove Press, 1982)
Out of print, but an updated version can be downloaded from http://www.claudesteiner.com/osp.htm

* 'the force that through the green fuse drives the flower': *Collected Poems*, Dylan Thomas (London: Dent, 1952), p 9

On the oppression of children:
* *The Drama of Being a Child*, Alice Miller (London: Virago, 1995)

* *Thou Shalt Not Be Aware: Society's betrayal of the child*, Alice Miller (London: Pluto, 1986)

On character and politics:
- *The Mass Psychology of Fascism*, Wilhelm Reich (New York: Farrar, Straus and Giroux, 1966)

A politically aware survey of various therapeutic approaches:
- *In Our Own Hands*, Sheila Ernst and Lucy Goodison (London: Women's Press, 1981)

On running therapy workshops on political issues:
- *Sitting in the Fire*, Arnold Mindell (Portland, OR: Lao Tse Press, 1995)

On psychotherapy and politics:
- *The Political Psyche*, Andrew Samuels (London: Routledge, 1993)
- *Psychotherapy and Politics*, Nick Totton (London: Sage, 2000)
- *The Politics of Psychotherapy*, Nick Totton, ed (Maidenhead: Open University Press, 2006)

An eloquent critique of the power relationships of therapy in general:
- *Against Therapy*, Jeffrey Masson (London: Fontana, 1990)

CHAPTER 10: PRIMAL PATTERNS

- *Realms of the Human Unconscious*, Stanislav Grof (New York: Dutton, 1976)
- *The Human Encounter with Death*, Stanislav Grof and Joan Halifax (London: Souvenir Press, 1978)
- *The Facts of Life*, RD Laing (London: Penguin, 1992)
- *The Voice of Experience*, RD Laing (Harmondsworth: Penguin, 1983)
- *The Ancestor Syndrome: Transgenerational psychotherapy and the hidden links in the family tree*, Anne Ancelin Schutzenberger (London: Routledge, 1998)

CHAPTER 11: COSMIC STREAMING

- *Cutting Through Spiritual Materialism*, Chögyam Trungpa (Boston: Shambhala, 1992)
- *Ether, God and Devil and Cosmic Superimposition*, Wilhelm Reich (New York: Farrar, Straus and Giroux, 1972)
- *The Cosmic Pulse of Life*, Trevor Constable (Suffolk: Neville Spearman, 1976)

Further Reading **159**

- *Orgone, Reich and Eros*, W Edward Mann (New York: Simon and Schuster, 1973)
- *Orgone Accumulator Handbook*, James Demeo (Ashland, OR: Natural Energy Works, 1992)
- Public Orgonomic Research Exchange, www.orgone.org
- *Needles of Stone*, Tom Graves (Girvan, Ayrshire: Grey House in the Woods, 2008)
- *Core Energetics*, Dr John Pierrakos (Mendocino, CA: Life Rhythm, 1998)
Another neo-Reichian synthesis, with a lot of material on auras and subtle energy.

CHAPTER 12: CONNECTIONS AND DIRECTIONS

- *Planet Medicine* (2nd ed, two vols), Richard Grossinger (Berkeley, CA: North Atlantic Books, 1995)
A vast and magnificent survey and analysis of alternative therapy and healing, with a lot of material on Reich and other body-oriented approaches.

On the various approaches we mention in this chapter:
- *The Reality Game*, John Rowan (London: Routledge and Kegan Paul, 1983)

- *The Red Book of Gestalt*, Gaie Huston (London: Rochester Foundation, 1995)

- *Bioenergetics*, Alexander Lowen (New York: Arkana, 1994)

- *Deep Bodywork and Personal Development*, Jack W Painter (self-published)
A new edition is said to be on the way; for this and other material see http://www.bodymindintegration.net/

- *Body Learning: An introduction to the Alexander Technique*, Michael Gelb (London: Aurum Press, 2004)

- *Embrace Tiger, Return to Mountain: Essence of T'ai Chi*, Al Huang (San Francisco: Celestial Arts, 1988)

- *The Potent Self*, Moshe Feldenkrais (San Francisco: Harper and Row, 1985)

- *Mindfulness-Based Cognitive Therapy*, Rebecca Crane (London: Routledge, 2008)

- *Rebirthing in the New Age*, Leonard Orr and Sondra Ray (San Francisco: Celestial Arts, 1977)

- *The Polarity Process: Energy as a healing art*, Franklyn Sills (Longmead, Dorset: Element, 1989)

- *Bone, Breath and Gesture: Practices of embodiment*, Don Hanlon Johnson, ed (Berkeley, CA: North Atlantic Books, 1995)
A fascinating collection of classic writings on body and movement work.

- *Despair and Empowerment in the Nuclear Age*, Joanna Macy (Philadelphia, PA: New Society, 1983)

Index

A

abuse 101, 118, 122, 131
   sexual 81, 82, 84
accumulators (see orgone
   accumulators)
Adler, Janet 150
adolescence 56, 154 (see also
   puberty)
affirmations 145
Alexander Technique 40, 144,
   153, 159
Alther, Lisa 157
anal block 75–8, 87
anus 51, 52, 62, 63, 89, 94
anxiety 25, 26, 32, 33, 38, 81,
   82, 83, 106, 140
   state, chronic 21
Aposhyan, Susan 156
Appignanesi, Richard 151
armour/ing 4, 15, 18, 19, 20,
   24, 25, 26, 28, 30, 53,
   54, 57, 62, 85, 100, 120,
   133, 134, 143, 151
   and character 57, 103, 105,
      111
   emotional 16
      energy and 11ff
   and illness 20
   in infants and children 131,
      133, 152
   muscle 99
   process of self- 28
association, free 142
assumptions 105, 106, 110,
   134, 145

Astington, Janet Wilde 155
asymmetrical, therapy relationship as 119
attachment 2, 3, 149
   theory 149
aura 69, 139, 159
Authentic Movement 4, 150
authority 57, 104, 118, 120
   figure 112

B

baby 13, 14, 36, 63, 67, 69,
   150, 155
   breathing 13
back 51, 61, 153
   and shoulders 54
   tension, lower 45, 46
Baker, Elsworth F 153
Bates, WH 153
Bean, Orson 157
belly 15
   segment 29, 45, 46–8
      armouring 48
      blocking 89
bioenergetics 143, 151, 154, 159
birth 34, 38, 86, 126, 127, 129,
   135, 139
   canal 126
   natural 130
   '-shaped experience' 127–30
birthing 128, 129
   experience 127, 130
   Re- 146, 160
Boadella, David 53, 150, 151,
   154

body
- -based emotional discharge techniques 156
- exercises 153
- -fantasies 130
- and movement work 160
- -oriented approaches 159
- -patterning 153
- psychotherapy 2, 3, 4, 19, 156, 157 (passim)

bodymind 12, 20, 22, 26, 27, 28, 30, 46, 53, 54, 57, 100, 101, 108, 130, 157
- armoured 57

bodywork 5, 7, 38, 97, 101, 102, 116, 143
- technique 107, 108

boundary/ies 17, 54, 67, 89, 124
- character 68, 69, 72, 83, 90, 94, 112, 135
- /crisis bridge 94
- /oral bridge 90-1
- therapeutic 110, 124

boundary character position 67-70, 82, 86, 90, 94, 112, 135

Bowlby, John 2, 149
Boyesen, Gerda 48
breastfeeding 36, 56, 70, 126
breath/ing 2, 12, 13, 14, 15, 17, 24, 25, 26, 41, 42, 43, 46, 48, 97, 98, 99, 100, 116, 128, 152, 160
- circular 128
- conscious connected 46, 146
- effects of armouring 18, 45, 60, 100, 101
- free 24, 25, 26, 142
- natural 13, 14
- over- 100
- pulsation of natural 13, 14

'bridge' character positions 90-3, 94
Buddhism 59, 136, 152
buttocks 51, 54, 76, 78, 87

C

capitalism 95
carer, compulsive 72
case histories 9, 156
centering 53-4, 154
chakras 138
change 5, 6, 7, 9, 21, 22, 57, 106, 121, 143
- emotional 144
character 95, 104, 112, 125, 150, 155-6
- armour/ing 57, 103, 105, 111
- combinations 92-3
- open 4
- and politics 158
- positions 4, 65, 85, 87-90, 112
  - boundary 67-70, 90, 94, 112, 135
  - control 73-5, 91
  - crisis 80-4, 88-90, 94, 112
  - holding 75-8, 91, 94
  - open 84-5
  - oral 70-3, 91, 112
  - summary of 86-8
  - thrusting 78-80, 91, 94
- rigid 91
- theory 156
chest segment 15, 40-3
- block 87
child 35
- sexuality 82
childhood 2, 24, 27, 154, 155
children 17, 36, 131
- oppression of 157
- experience of 155

Index **163**

Chögyam Trungpa 21, 40, 135, 152, 153, 158
client, being a 109, 114–16
cloudbuster 7, 137
COEX systems 126, 127
Cognitive Behavioural Therapy (CBT) 144
Cognitive Therapy 159
Conger, John 156
connective tissue 61, 143
Constable, Trevor 158
contact 3, 43, 67, 68, 74, 96, 97, 102, 110, 111, 112, 123, 137
   repression of 32
   resistance to 104
control
   character 4, 74, 75
   /holding bridge 91
   oral/, bridge 92–3
control character position 73–5, 87, 91
core 58, 60, 62, 96
   of a human being is loving 114
   nature 59
Corrington, Robert S 151
counter-transference 109, 111
Crane, Rebecca 159
craniosacral rhythm 12
crisis
   /boundary bridge 94
   holding/, bridge 94
crisis character position 80–4, 88–90, 94, 112

D

Damasio, Antonio 30, 153
defence 38, 54, 58, 104, 110, 142
   armouring as 18, 57, 127
   character as system of 104, 112
   structures of 142
   transference as 111, 112, 113
defending 57
Demeo, James 159
denial 15, 17, 23, 27, 66, 145
Denman, Chess 152
development
   cognitive 74, 89
   early years 75, 76, 126, 132
   embryonic and foetal 155
   phases 61, 62, 63, 67, 81, 83, 132
   process 56, 63
   threshold of 57, 65, 132
diaphragm 14, 43–6, 48, 54, 101
   block 94
discharge 23, 25
   emotion 11, 23, 35, 59, 64, 156
   tension 3, 24
Donaldson, Margaret 155
Dychtwald, Ken 153

E

earth energy 50, 66, 139
ecology 5, 122
ego 16, 21, 38, 79, 135
   psychology 156
   'spastic' 133
Embodied-Relational Therapy 156
embodiment 2, 38, 139, 143
embryo 29, 61
embryonic and foetal development 155
emotion/s 11, 12, 13, 15, 17, 22, 23, 24, 27, 28, 33, 34, 35, 36, 37, 38, 40, 43, 44, 48, 49, 99, 101, 102–5, 152 (see also feelings)

negative 114
physical illness and 84
emotional
　armouring 16
　attitudes, fossilised 107
　change 144
　rational basis of 22
　secondary 60
　tone, rigid 18
emotionally
　cold 14
　toxic environments 19
energy 2, 107, 151
　and armour 11ff
　-exchange segments 65, 75, 95
　life 2, 5, 7, 11, 12, 14, 26, 97, 134, 137
　pulsating exchange of 24
　splits 14
　split-off 16
　Stream 8, 9, 10
Epstein, Mark 152
Ernst, Sheila 150
erogenous zones 65
Evison, Rose 152
exercises 154
eye segment 30–4
　armouring 30, 31, 32, 34, 51, 107
　block 86

F

facing 53–4, 66, 154
family 119, 131
　abuses of children 131
　influences 95
　themes 131, 132
fear 16, 22, 32, 39, 41, 68, 111, 118
feeding 17, 36, 56, 62, 67, 70–2, 87
feeling/s 12, 14, 15, 16, 22, 23, 99 (see also emotions)
　expressed through eyes 33
　gut 44, 46
feet 49, 50, 51, 52, 53
Feitis, Rosemary 154
Feldenkrais, Moshe 159
　Method 144
Fine, Anne 154
Frank, Ruella 157
free association 142
Freud, Emma 154
Freud, Sigmund 2, 126, 151
　on the ego 151

G

gagging
　and coughing 35, 38
　and retching 46
Gelb, Michael 153, 159
gender 80, 81, 88, 122, 132
　roles 82, 84
genital/s 51, 62, 63, 88
　area 51
　character 4, 84, 150
　revenge 79
Gerhardt, Sue 149
Gestalt Therapy 142, 157
Goldhawk, Tessa 152
Gonzalez, German 150
Goodison, Lucy 158
Graves, Tom 159
Grof, Stanislav 126, 158
Grossinger, Richard 155, 159
ground, contact with the 50, 52
groundedness 47, 50
grounding 53–4, 57, 76, 87, 129, 139, 143, 154
　over- 66
　under- 66, 69
groups 53, 116–17

H

Hakomi method 150, 155
   therapy 4
Haldane, Sean 156
Halifax, Joan 158
Hay, Louise 152
heart 4, 32
   centre 75
   segment 29, 39, 40-3, 62, 65, 66, 89
      armouring 42, 43
      block 73-5
Heckler, Richard 156
holding
   /crisis bridge 94
   /thrusting bridge 91
holding character position 65, 75-8, 81, 87, 89, 91, 94
Holmes, Jeremy 149
homosexual 8
   anti-, stance 8
Horobin, Richard 152
House, Richard 149
Huang, Al 159
human nature 9, 39
humanistic psychology 142
Huston, Gaie 159
hyperventilation 100
'hysteric' 80, 83, 84

I

illness 84, 142, 152
   armouring and 20
imagery 107, 108, 130
   body 90
infancy 67, 132, 155
infantile feelings 71
involuntary 26
   breathing 26, 46
   muscles 62

J

Jacobs, Michael 156, 157
Jansson, Tove 154
jaw and mouth segment 34-7
   armouring 36, 38
   block 70, 87
Johnson, Don Hanlon 160
Johnson, Stephen M 156

K

Keleman, Stanley 53, 151, 154
Kurtz, Ron 153, 155

L

Laing, Ronald D 69, 156, 158
Lao Tsu 141
legs 14, 29, 49, 50-3
Levine, Peter 152
libido 2
life energy 2, 5, 7, 11, 12, 14, 20, 51, 97, 107, 108, 134, 137, 138 (see also orgone)
   splits 14
loving 18, 20, 58, 59, 114, 120
Lowen, Alexander 50, 94, 143, 151, 153, 154, 155, 159
Lowen, Leslie 153, 154

M

machismo 79, 94
Macnaughton, Ian 152
Macy, Joanna 147, 160
Mairowitz, David Zane 150
Mann, William E 151, 159
martial arts and Reichian perspectives 156
Masson, Jeffrey 158
men, thrusting character encouraged in 79

Middle Layer 58, 59, 60
Miller, Alice 157
Mindell, Amy 150
Mindell, Arnold 4, 114, 150, 157, 158
   Process Work 4
money 118, 123, 124
Mossner, Heidrun 150
Mother Earth 50
mouth (see jaw and mouth)
mucus 11, 38
muscle/s
   armour (see armour/ing)
   flaccid 16, 21, 152
   tension 12, 15, 28, 52, 97

N

Nazis 7
neck segment, throat and (see throat and neck segment)
neuroscience 3, 19, 30, 149, 153, 157
Nietzsche, Friedrich 06
nose/anus relationship 52

O

Oedipal stage 132
Oedipus Complex 81
Ogdon, Pat 152
open character position 84–5
oral
   blocking 72
   boundary/, bridge 90
   /control bridge 91
oral character position 70–3, 87, 91, 112
Oranur experiment 7
orgasm 24, 25, 27, 138
   reflex 26, 52
orgone 11, 276, 107, 136, 137, 138, 139, 147, 151, 157, 159
   accumulator 7, 136, 137
   cloudmelter 137
   device, human being is 108
Orr, Leonard 160

P

pain in bodywork 101
Painter, Jack W 159
Pallaro, Patriazia 150
'past life memories' 130
patriarchy 27, 80, 84, 94, 95, 119, 122, 134
pelvic
   block 78–80, 87, 88
      against opening 80–4
   relaxation 25
   segment 49–53, 60
      armouring 49, 51
Perls, Fritz 142
personality 58, 77
   armoured 120
   three layers of 155
   types 156
personhood, different styles of 156
Pert, Candace 153
Phillips, Adam 155
phobias 50, 145
Pierrakos, John 159
play/ing 63, 73, 74, 85, 88
   games 83
pleasure 24, 25, 26, 27, 63, 79, 81, 84
   erotic 27, 34, 79
   frustrated 38, 62
   lost 18
Polarity Therapy 146, 160
politics 23, 27, 158
   issues, therapy workshops on 158
politically aware survey 158
Postle, Denis 149
Postural Integration 143–4

power 16, 18, 42, 63, 76, 81, 100, 101, 118ff
   -for 119, 124, 157
   issues 116
   -over 60, 119, 124, 157
   patriarchal 27, 94
   relationships of therapy 110, 111, 112, 118, 119, 158
Prestera, Hector 153
primal
   impulses 58
   interactions 34
   patterns 125ff, 155
   terror 44
Process Oriented Psychotherapy 157
Process Work 4, 150
projections 110
Proulx, Annie 154
psoas muscle 49, 52
psychic 68, 69, 86, 133, 134
   experience 135,
   powers 135
psychoanalysis 5, 7, 94, 110, 126, 142
   Freudian 110
psychopathic 74
psychotherapy
   body, varieties of 21, 156, 157
   and politics 158
puberty
   first 81, 82
   second 81, 82
pulsation 12, 24
   of natural breathing 13, 14

R

Raknes, Ola 151
Ray, Sondra 160
Rebirthing 146, 164
rectus abdominis muscles 47, 48

regression 63, 125
regulation
   self- 18, 60, 62, 75–7, 122
   therapy 1, 2
Reich, Peter 150
Reich, Wilhelm 1, 2, 3, 5, 6, 7–8, 9, 14, 19, 25, 26, 28, 49, 58, 65, 68, 79, 97, 118, 119, 122, 136, 139, 143, 146, 149, 150, 151, 152, 155, 156, 158, 159
   intellectual autobiography 151
   origins in psychoanalysis 151
   work and ideas 151
Reichian
   bodywork 5, 97 (passim)
   character theory 156
   martial arts and 156
   therapy 157 (passim)
      Jungian's experience of 157
      person's experience of 157
   training in 8
relationship 141
   and character positions 70
   with the ground 53
   long-term 27
   therapy 97, 101, 109–13, 118, 119, 123, 141
   (see also transference)
relaxation 1, 17, 21, 100
release 12, 33, 35, 42, 48, 52, 60, 67, 99, 101
   sexual 24, 25, 49
remedial
   therapies 97, 144
   work 144, 145
repression 45, 59, 66, 99, 147
   of contact 32
resistance 23, 24, 35, 111, 143
   to feeling 23, 103, 111

revenge 74
  genital 79
Rilke, Rainer Maria 86, 125
Rolfing 143, 154
Rothschild, Babette 152
Rowan, John 159

S

Samuels, Andrew 158
scarcity, myth of 119
Schultz, R Louis 154
Schutzenberger, Anne Ancelin 158
Scott Peck, M 155
segment/s 18, 19, 28, 37, 66, 89, 95, 153 (see also individual segments: eye, jaw and throat, neck, heart, waist, belly, pelvic)
  seven 29
self
  -armouring, process of 28
  -contempt 70
  -expression, spontaneous 1
    blocked 94
  heal 10
  -help (peer therapy) 96
sex 7, 24, 27, 49, 50, 122
  and surrender 24–7
sexism 122
sexual
  abuse 81, 82, 84
  energy 81
  excitement 25, 81
  release 24, 25, 49
sexuality 25, 27, 49, 81
  children's 78, 81, 82
Shamanism 136
shame 23, 76, 121
Sharaf, Myron 150
Sills, Franklyn 160
skull, base of the 30, 31, 39
social conditions 7

sound, making 34, 38, 99, 100, 101
'Spastic I' 16–18, 21, 25, 26, 49, 133
Spiegelman, J Marvin 157
spiritual 69, 133 (see also psychic)
  materialism 21, 135
spirituality 34, 135
spontaneity 1, 21, 25, 26, 45, 107, 112, 114
Steiner, Claude 157
Stern, Daniel N 155
sternocleidomastoid muscles 37, 39, 48
streaming 26, 81, 132
  cosmic 133ff
stress 21
  -related ailments 46, 83
supernatural 133 (see also psychic, spiritual)
Surface layer 58, 59

T

T'ai Chi 144, 159
tension 1, 3, 13, 15, 17, 21, 25, 28, 31, 36, 46
therapeutic work, accounts of 156
therapist, being a 96, 97, 103, 104, 105, 111, 113, 114
therapy 96ff
  empowered by 3
  goals of 6, 19, 95, 106, 113–14
  group 116–17, 124
  relationship 109–13
    power in (see power)
  resistance in 104, 105
  sessions, peer 96, 116–17
  state regulation of 1, 2, 149
  therapist in 103, 115
thinking 32, 33, 34, 105, 106

Index

as an escape 33
positive 144, 145
Thomas, Dylan 119, 157
thought 105–7
throat and neck segment 29, 35, 37–40, 46, 62
armouring 38–40
thrusting
character,
encouraged in men 79
position 78–80, 91, 94
/crisis bridge 94
thrusting character position 78–80, 83, 87, 91, 94, 112
toilet training 17, 75, 76, 126
Totton, Nick 149, 150, 151, 156, 158
training in Reichian therapy 8
transference 109, 110, 111, 112, 113, 117, 119, 139, 141, 142, 147
relationship 110
Trapido, Barbara 154
trauma/s 2, 3, 4, 19–20, 85, 142, 146, 149, 152
chronic 20

U

umbilical cord 48, 54, 56, 129
unconscious 15, 45, 46, 126, 131, 142, 145
blocking 15, 51, 60, 103
wisdom 144

V

visualisation 108, 145, 149
voice 34, 39, 40, 99, 100

W

waist segment 43–6
armouring 46

walking 49, 50
Walker, Moira 157
weaning 36, 70, 71
West, William 8, 9, 45, 151
Wilson, Jacqueline 154
Winnicott, Donald Woods 155
Winterson, Jeanette 154
women 48, 68, 80, 82
therapy for 157
Woolf, Virginia 154
Wordsworth, William 154

Y

yearning 66, 74, 83, 88, 89 (see also oral character position)
block 68, 81

Z

Zarate, Oscar 151

WILD THERAPY
Undomesticating inner and outer worlds

Nick Totton

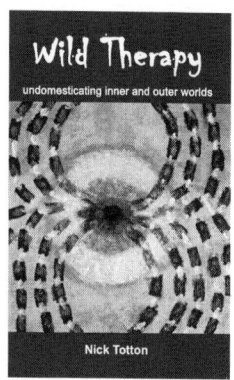

ISBN 978-1-906254-36-0

Therapy is by nature wild; but a lot of it at the moment is rather tame. This book tries to shift the balance back towards wildness, by connecting therapy with ecological thinking, seeing each species, each being, and each person inherently and profoundly linked to each other. Therapists have always tried to help people tolerate the anxiety of not being in control of our feelings, our thoughts, our body, our future. Human efforts to control the world are well on the way to wrecking it through environmental collapse: the more we try to control things, the further out of balance we push them. Nick Totton describes a mode of being present in all cultures, 'Wild Mind', and explores how this can be supported through a 'wild therapy', bringing together a wide range of already-existing ideas and practices, which may have a role to play in creating a new culture that can live well on the earth without damaging ourselves and other beings.

> Nick Totton's 'Wild Therapy' is a call from nature to rediscover the earth and relationship to the universe. Totton's 'wildness' is a breath of fresh air, freeing therapies and cultures to live closer to the Tao. Read, dream, and be moved by his book! Arnold Mindell, author of 'Processmind'

CONTENTS: 1 Wild Roots, 2 Wild Complexity, 3 In and Out of the Wilderness, 4 Wild Mind, 5 Domesticating Wild Mind, 6 Wildness Under Control, 7 Wild/Human, 8 Wild Therapies, 9 Wild Therapy, 10 Living Wild

Order direct www.pccs-books.co.uk   +44(0)1600 891509

Not a Tame Lion

Writings on therapy and its social and political contexts

Nick Totton

ISBN 978 1 906254 48 3

Collected together for the first time, articles and chapters from Nick Totton's writing over many years. Discussing the politics of psychotherapy; his themes include democracy, equality, professionalisation and regulation, pluralism, boundaries and ecopsychology. A collection that will make you think. As Nick says: '... this collection of direct or implicit arguments about the wild nature of therapy, and its intrinsic unsuitability for domestication, seem to me well worth assembling.' (Introduction, p. xi)

In four parts:
Part One: Professionalisation and Regulation
Part Two: The Nature of Therapy
Part Three: Therapy in the World
Part Four: Ecopsychology and Embodiment

Order direct www.pccs-books.co.uk   +44(0)1600 891509